Book Loan

Complementary and Alternative
Medicine: Structures and Safeguards

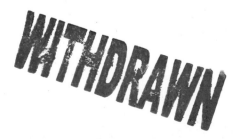

0415351626

This book forms part of the core text for the Open University course K221 Perspectives on Complementary and Alternative Medicine and is related to other materials available to students, including two more texts also published by Routledge:

- *Perspectives on Complementary and Alternative Medicine* (Book 1)

- *Perspectives on Complementary and Alternative Medicine: A Reader* (Set Book).

If you are interested in studying this course, or related courses, please write to the Information Officer, Faculty of Health and Social Care, The Open University, Walton Hall, Milton Keynes MK7 6AA, UK.

Details are also given on the web page at www.open.ac.uk

Complementary and Alternative Medicine: Structures and Safeguards

Edited by Geraldine Lee-Treweek, Tom Heller, Hilary MacQueen,
Julie Stone and Sue Spurr (The Open University)

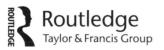 in association with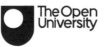

This book forms part of an Open University course K221 Perspectives on Complementary and Alternative Medicine. Details of this and other Open University courses can be obtained from the Course Information and Advice Centre, PO Box 724, The Open University, Milton Keynes MK7 6ZS, United Kingdom: tel. +44 (0)1908 653231; e-mail ces-gen@open.ac.uk

Alternatively, you may visit the Open University website at www.open.ac.uk where you can learn more about the wide range of courses and packs offered at all levels by The Open University.

To purchase this publication or other components of Open University courses, contact Open University Worldwide Ltd, The Open University, Walton Hall, Milton Keynes MK7 6AA, United Kingdom: tel. +44 (0)1908 858785; fax +44 (0)1908 858787; e-mail ouwenq@open.ac.uk; website www.ouw.co.uk

First published 2005 by Routledge
2 Park Square, Milton Park, Abingdon OX14 4RN
Simultaneously published in the USA and Canada by Routledge
270 Madison Avenue, New York, NY 10016
Routledge is an imprint of the Taylor & Francis Group

Edited, designed and typeset by The Open University.

Printed and bound in the United Kingdom by The Alden Group (Oxford).

ISBN 0-415-351-626 (hbk)

ISBN 0-415-351-634 (pbk)

1.1

307240B/k221b2prelimsi1.1

Contents

Contributors

Geraldine Lee-Treweek is a sociologist of health and illness and was a Lecturer in Health Studies at The Open University until autumn 2004. Her main field of specialism is complementary and unorthodox healing, in particular CAM therapeutic relationships, the experience of long-term users of CAM and the professionalisation of modalities. She also has long-standing interests in chronic illness and disability, trust and belief in contemporary society, social gerontology and the sociology of unexplained phenomena.

Tom Heller is a general practitioner in a deprived area of Sheffield. His practice is associated with the integration of complementary and alternative forms of practice alongside orthodox medical approaches. For the last 20 years he has also been a Senior Lecturer in the Faculty of Health and Social Care at The Open University and involved in the production of a series of health-related courses.

Hilary MacQueen is a Senior Lecturer in Health Sciences in the Faculty of Science, and Director of the Health Sciences Programme at The Open University. She trained as a microbiologist and cell biologist. Her current research investigates the role of dietary fat in modulating the inflammatory immune response.

Julie Stone is Deputy Director of the Council for Healthcare Regulatory Excellence. She was previously a lecturer in health care ethics and law, teaching pre- and post-registration health care practitioners across a wide range of conventional and CAM professions. A lawyer by training, Julie has advised many CAM bodies on ethical and legal responsibilities and has contributed to policy initiatives in the CAM arena both nationally and internationally. Julie has written and lectured extensively on legal, ethical and regulatory aspects of complementary and alternative medicine. Her books include: *Complementary Medicine and the Law* (1996, Oxford University Press) with Joan Matthews; *An Ethical Framework for Complementary and Alternative Therapists* (2002, Routledge); and *Psychotherapy and the Law* (2004, Whurr) with Peter Jenkins and Vincent Keter.

Sue Spurr is a Course Manager in the Faculty of Health and Social Care at The Open University, working on health-related courses. She is a qualified teacher of science and biology and is currently training to become a shiatsu practitioner.

Lorraine Williams originally trained as a nurse and midwife and has been a practising midwife in London and Oxford for several years. She is a sociology graduate and has lectured in social sciences and health studies to health and social care practitioners in a number of further and higher education institutions. She is currently working at the Prince of Wales's Foundation for Integrated Health as education and training development manager. Here she has been involved in writing and contributing to journal articles and professional and public guidance materials on the regulation, education and practice of complementary and integrated health care in the UK.

Professor Mike Saks is Pro Vice Chancellor at the University of Lincoln. He was formerly Dean of the Faculty of Health and Community Studies at De Montfort University. He has published extensively on professionalisation, health care and complementary and alternative medicine and given many presentations at national and international conferences. His latest books include *Regulating the Health Professions*, *Complementary Medicine: Challenge and Change* and *Orthodox and Alternative Medicine: Professionalization, Politics and Health Care*. He has been a member and chair of numerous NHS committees and has served on a range of national groups on complementary and alternative medicine, including the NHS research and development capacity building committee for this area. He is a member of the Executive of the International Sociological Association Research Committee on Professional Groups and the editorial team for the new international journal *Knowledge, Work and Society*, as well as the current Chair of the Research Council for Complementary Medicine.

Phil Nicholls studied sociology at Nottingham University, graduating in 1977. After completing a postgraduate certificate in education at the University of Leicester, he returned to Nottingham to begin work on his doctoral thesis. This focused on the history of homeopathic medicine in the UK, and was awarded in 1984. He has worked in the Department of Sociology at Staffordshire University since 1979, where he is now a principal lecturer, teaching the sociology of health and medicine and comparative social structure. Since publishing *Homoeopathy and the Medical Profession* (Croom Helm, 1988), he has continued to research and publish in the area of complementary and alternative medicine.

Sheena Murdoch has over 20 years' experience of conducting social research and acting as a research adviser. She has extensive experience of teaching, training and writing about social research methodologies and methods, specialising in qualitative research. She holds a BA (Hons), an MSc, a PgDip (Research Methods for the Social Sciences) and a PhD in Sociology.

Andrew Vickers is a research methodologist and statistician who has focused on complementary and alternative medicine for much of his career. He received his Bachelor's degree in the History and Philosophy of Science from the University of Cambridge and his doctorate in Clinical Medicine from the University of Oxford. He has been an investigator on numerous clinical trials and systematic reviews of complementary therapies, including a study of acupuncture for headache that is among the largest randomised trials of acupuncture ever conducted. He has also conducted considerable statistical and methodological research, with a particular emphasis on randomised trials with quality-of-life outcomes. Dr Vickers now works at Memorial Sloan-Kettering Cancer Center in New York where he has appointments in the Departments of Medicine, Biostatistics,

Urology and Public Health (Weill Cornell Medical College). Dr Vickers' most recent methodological research has centred on medical prediction.

Dick Heller is a physician and an epidemiologist and is currently Professor of Public Health at the University of Manchester. He spent 17 years working in Australia, where he was involved in developments in evidence-based medicine and its teaching in Australia and the developing world. His new unit in Manchester – the Evidence for Population Health Unit – has the mission to build a public health counterpart to evidence-based medicine. His research interests involve the development of measures to describe the population impact of risks and benefits. He has also been involved in developing a new, fully online Masters course: Masters in Population Health Evidence (www.mphe.man.ac.uk).

Gavin Yamey was recently appointed Senior Editor at *PLoS Medicine*, a leading international medical journal published by the Public Library of Science (PLoS). PLoS is an international non-profit organisation dedicated to making the world's biomedical literature a public resource. Gavin has a BA (First Class Honours) in Physiological Sciences from Oxford University (1991) and became an MD in 1994. He was awarded Membership of the Royal College of Physicians (UK) in 1997. In 1999 he joined the *British Medical Journal* (BMJ) and became an Assistant Editor. In 2000 he was appointed Deputy Editor of the *Western Journal of Medicine*, a primary care journal based in San Francisco. He has published several hundred articles on health and medicine in scholarly journals, magazines, newspapers and books, including an acclaimed five-part investigative series about the World Health Organization (published in the BMJ in 2000). He has been a public radio commentator, and has run training workshops for medical journalists and editors in Barcelona and Addis Ababa. He has been a consultant to the World Health Organization and The Open University (UK). He lives in San Francisco.

Elaine Weatherley-Jones, PhD, Chartered Psychologist and Registered Homeopath, is Senior Research Fellow in the Health Services Research section of the School of Health and Related Research at the University of Sheffield. Her current research is funded through the Department of Health's Capacity Building Award Scheme in Complementary and Alternative Medicine. As part of this award, she intends to describe how people experience the homeopathic consultation. She has published research on a trial of homeopathic treatment for chronic fatigue syndrome and a critique of the randomised, controlled, placebo trial in homeopathy. While most of her time is spent researching, she also spends some time each week in clinical practice as a homeopath. She has worked locally in a drop-in centre for injecting drug users, a centre offering complementary therapies to people living with cancer and the minor injuries section of the local accident and emergency service in a Sheffield NHS hospital and has recently started work in an NHS community homeopathy clinic. All of these clinics offer patients treatment free of charge.

Dione Hills, BSc. (Hons), PhD, has been involved in the evaluation of innovative approaches to health and social care provision for over 20 years. After seven years as a researcher with the Department of Health, she joined the Tavistock Institute as a Senior Researcher/Consultant. In this role she has been involved in the evaluation of several programmes, including major initiatives in the area of community care, support for disabled people, and health education at a community level. Currently, this includes the programme-wide evaluation of the Healthy Living Centre Initiatives (community health interventions to address health inequalities). Previous programme evaluations include the European Commission programme for equal rights and integration of disabled people (HELIOS II) and the DSS/DfEE programme New Deal for Disabled People, Innovative Schemes. A major theme in her research is the involvement and empowerment of service users, particularly related to excluded groups. As scientific adviser to the Department of Health's 'Health in Partnership' research programme, Dione recently contributed to an overview report on 12 new research projects concerned with engaging patients, carers and the public in health care decision making. She is currently project manager for the Department of Health and New Opportunities Fund Evaluation of the Healthy Living Centres programme.

Acknowledgements

Grateful acknowledgement is made to the following sources for permission to reproduce material in this book.

Chapter 1

Photographs

p. 11: © Sheila Terry/Science Photo Library; p. 18: © James Randi/Associated Press.

Chapter 2

Photographs

p. 37: courtesy of Sue Spurr; p. 40: © Alix/Phanie(PHN)/Rex features.

Chapter 4

Photographs

p. 76 (top left, top and bottom centre, and right): © Alamy Images; p. 76 (bottom left): © PhotoDisc Europe Limited; p. 84: © The Wellcome Trust; p. 90: © Sally and Richard Greenhill; p. 96: by kind permission of the Harry Edwards Healing Sanctuary Ltd, www.harryedwards.org.uk.

Chapter 5

Photographs

p. 104 and p. 108: © Science Photo Library; p. 118: © Association Jacques Benveniste pour la Recherché, http://jacques.benveniste.org.

Chapter 6

Photographs

p. 130: © Mary Evans Picture Library; p. 133 (left and right): © Science Photo Library; p. 146: © Cartoon Stock, www.CartoonStock.com; p. 148: © Mauro Fermariello/Science Photo Library.

Chapter 7

Photographs

p. 159: University of Toronto Archives and Records Management Services; p. 160: © Science Photo Library; p. 165: Block, J. R. (2002) 'Ambiguous figures and figure-ground images', *Seeing Double*, Taylor and Francis Books Ltd.

Chapter 8

Photographs

p. 197: © Science Photo Library; p. 200: © Sally and Richard Greenhill; p. 210: © Science Photo Library.

Text

Box 8.6: adapted from O'Meara et al. (2002) 'Effective health care', *NHS Centre for Reviews and Dissemination*, Vol. 7, No. 3. Reproduced by permission of the University of York.

Chapter 9

Text

Box 9.5: adapted from Monk, J. and Chaplin, S. (2002) *Complementary Health in Partnerships (CHIPS) Evaluation Report – Update*, Community at Heart.

Front cover

Photograph

Copyright © Science Photo Library

Introduction

There has been a rapid growth in the popularity of complementary and alternative medicine (CAM) throughout the UK over recent decades (Ong and Banks, 2003). This book focuses on CAM as a dynamic and emerging field and, specifically, addresses current issues and debates around safeguards, standards and efficacy. The book is premised on the idea that, while the growth of CAM represents increased choice (for consumers, practitioners and health care providers), it also raises issues about how individuals can use CAM safely and with confidence. This book considers how standards of practice are created and maintained, the ways in which CAM practitioners are working towards professional standing and recognition, and the different ways of researching and evaluating CAM. These issues are not important only to CAM: increasing regulation, protection of the public, monitoring of individual practitioners and professional standards and a focus on the need for evidence of efficacy are features in many other spheres within western societies (Beck, 1992). In these societies people have become increasingly aware of risks that might arise from other aspects of their lives and they want to manage those risks through understanding the treatments on offer and making informed decisions based on 'evidence' and the latest research. On a broader level, there are also other groups who need good quality evidence and research to inform their work, such as orthodox health and social care professionals, managers in public and private health services, policymakers and CAM practitioners or organisations. This book explores how safeguards, standards, professional development and efficacy overlap and interact in the dynamic and constantly changing world of CAM.

Until recently in the UK, CAM was presented as something out of the ordinary: a group of diverse therapies and ideas about the world that were antithetical to 'rational' thinking and orthodox approaches to health (BMA, 1989). This view has (at least partially) been replaced by a genuine interest in CAM by the same orthodox establishments (BMA, 1993; General Medical Council, 2001). This book begins by exploring the way in which the definition of some knowledge as marginal, unscientific and/or irrational impacts on how that knowledge is seen and valued within society in general. The first chapter promotes the idea that knowledge is political in the sense that it is not neutral; what is often presented as fact, truth or indeed humbug is often labelled for particular partisan reasons. Examples are used to demonstrate how debates about knowledge have affected CAM: in relation to disputes with other forms of knowledge (in particular science); in relation to disagreements within CAM disciplines; and when conflicts arise among different CAM disciplines. Finally, the issue of fraud and deception is addressed and the reader is asked to critically consider whether such terms are usually deployed by one group to negatively define the knowledge of others, or whether they are necessary terms to describe untried and untested knowledge. The context is set for thinking about safeguards, standards and structures by questioning how or whether legitimate knowledge can be objectively defined.

Next some of the safeguards and structures within CAM are examined by focusing on educational development and standards. The notion of 'charismatic training' (Cant, 2005) is used to discuss how some CAM modalities have developed from a model of individual teachers taking students through their CAM training using personal charisma and drive. This form of teaching has been largely superseded by more formal training and educational structures that have developed in most popular CAM therapies. However, education and training in CAM are very diverse and in many disciplines formalised learning is not necessarily the only appropriate method of learning. This is especially the case in relation to CAM therapies that originated in cultures where a higher value is placed on oral history and personalised forms of knowledge transmission than in the West. Current developments in CAM education and training are discussed to give a view of the changing landscape of this area. These developments include the creation of National Occupational Standards, continuing professional development (CPD), and the trend towards the familiarisation of orthodox health care practitioners in CAM during their training.

Regulation of health care work is needed in order to safeguard standards and protect the public. The term 'regulation' relates to the ways in which groups organise, structure and manage themselves or are regulated by higher authorities, such as the state. There is considerable diversity in how different disciplines are regulated in CAM (Stone, 2002). Chapter 3 explains that some groups, such as osteopaths and chiropractors, have decided to use statutory self-regulation (SSR), which means they develop in such a way that the state protects them through statute. It is now illegal in the UK for practitioners to define themselves as osteopaths unless they are registered with the requisite regulatory body – the General Osteopathic Council. While osteopaths and chiropractors have taken this route, other CAM modalities self-regulate and yet others remain apparently unregulated in any discernible way. The field of CAM is a dynamic and changing setting in terms of regulation. The reader is introduced to the key issues and debates and the reasons why CAM groups might choose particular regulatory paths.

Professionalisation is the process through which an occupation is developed so that it becomes recognised as a profession by the state and by society in general. Chapter 4 examines the ways in which professionalisation has been understood by a variety of social scientific perspectives. It then uses one perspective – the neo-Weberian approach – to explore in depth how CAM professions have developed since the 1960s. While professionalisation may outwardly appear to be a disjointed process, the protection of sectional occupational interests is often at the core of professional development (Saks, 2005).

Chapter 5 brings together some of the key themes of Part 1 of this book by examining one popular CAM modality: homeopathy. This is classified as one of the 'Big Five' most popular and highly organised CAM therapies in the UK (House of Lords, 2000). It is practised by medical practitioners who have had further training (medical homeopaths), by practitioners who have trained but are not medically qualified (lay homeopaths), and by individuals when they purchase over-the-counter remedies to use at home. The knowledge bases and philosophical precepts of homeopathy are explained as well as those educational structures, regulation and professionalisation issues relating to homeopathy in the UK. Homeopathy raises some fundamental questions about what happens when a CAM modality has a view of the world that is deeply 'unscientific' when seen from the perspective of mainstream science. Of particular importance is the way in which labels of 'fraud' or 'quackery' have been applied to homeopathy, despite its popularity and use both in the UK and worldwide. The reader's attention is drawn to matters of evidence and efficacy and the demands on CAM practitioners that they should be able to demonstrate their efficacy, often using orthodox scientific methods.

The second part of this book addresses the core themes of evidence and efficacy in CAM and within the sphere of orthodox medicine. Although the randomised controlled trial is often considered to be the 'gold standard' for scientific research, many other approaches are currently being used by CAM researchers. In some instances, research uses qualitative or small-scale case study methods, which seek to understand the user's experience of CAM use, rather than just the outcome of using a particular therapy in isolation. Chapters 6 to 9 emphasise how the use of the full spectrum of methods can develop an evidence base that will take CAM forward in the 21st century.

The focus so far in this book is on CAM therapies and CAM practitioners. However, Chapter 6 takes the opportunity to look closely at orthodox medical practice. In what ways are the issues within orthodox medical practice similar to, or different from, those that have been examined within the world of CAM? In particular, this chapter sheds light on the practice of 'evidence-based medicine' and discusses many of the problems inherent in attempting to use the scientific method to help individuals in all their complexity. The placebo effect is explored and how it may be a valuable part of orthodox medical approaches, as well as possibly featuring within CAM approaches.

Chapters 7 to 9 look in considerable depth at the ways in which CAM interventions can be subjected to research and evaluation. Using a series of case studies, they explore many of the current methods that are used to provide additional 'evidence' that will illuminate how CAM is currently practised.

The future for CAM appears to be linked to the development of research and the accumulation of evidence that relates to efficacy. The drive for such research often comes from policy makers and those who want to see greater integration of CAM into orthodox health and social care settings. However, consumers of CAM are also becoming increasingly aware of the need to minimise risks and they may well become another driving force, insisting on safeguards, standards and structures in the therapies they use. CAM certainly does provide challenges for developing research programmes that will answer questions about effectiveness. In particular, philosophical issues around holism or different notions of how health and wellbeing are achieved can provide challenges for people who want to develop research programmes that will illuminate these critical issues.

Geraldine Lee-Treweek, Tom Heller and Sue Spurr, The Open University, February 2005

References

Beck, U. (1992) *Risk Society: Towards a New Modernity* (originally pub. 1986, trans. by Mark Ritter, with an Introduction by Scott Lash and Brian Wynne), London, Sage Publications.

British Medical Association (BMA) (1989) *Alternative Therapy: Report of the Board of Science and Education*, London, BMA.

British Medical Association (BMA) (1993) *Complementary Medicine: New Approaches to Good Practice*, London, BMA.

Cant, S. (2005) 'From charismatic teaching to professional training: the legitimation of knowledge and the creation of trust in homeopathy and chiropractic', in Lee-Treweek, G., Heller, T., Spurr, S., MacQueen, H. and Katz, J. (eds) *Perspectives on Complementary and Alternative Medicine: A Reader*, pp. 222–30, Abingdon, Routledge/The Open University (K221 Set Book).

General Medical Council (2001) *Good Medical Practice. Duties and Responsibilities of Doctors*, London, GMC.

House of Lords (2000) Select Committee on Science and Technology's Sixth Report, *Complementary and Alternative Medicine*, London, The Stationery Office.

Ong, C. and Banks, B. (2003) *Complementary and Alternative Medicine: The Consumer Perspective*, London, The Prince of Wales's Foundation for Integrated Health.

Saks, M. (2005) 'Regulating complementary and alternative medicine: the case of acupuncture', in Lee-Treweek, G., Heller, T., Spurr, S., MacQueen, H. and Katz, J. (eds) *Perspectives on Complementary and Alternative Medicine: A Reader*, pp. 252–9, Abingdon, Routledge/The Open University (K221 Set Book).

Stone, J. (2002) *An Ethical Framework for Complementary and Alternative Therapies*, London, Routledge.

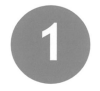

CAM Organisation: Safety and Standards

Edited by Tom Heller and Geraldine Lee-Treweek

Chapter 1 Knowledge, names, fraud and trust

Geraldine Lee-Treweek

Contents

AIMS

- To understand how knowledge competes for authenticity and legitimacy in social life and, in particular, the way this operates in CAM.
- To give an insight into the political nature of name-calling and blaming within CAM and between CAM and other forms of knowledge.
- To examine the notion and label of fraud and deception in relation to CAM therapies.

1.1 Introduction

In today's society there are increasing numbers of individuals or groups of people who claim to have knowledge that can help in health and wellbeing. On the one hand, this can be seen as a positive trend that allows people to make choices. On the other hand, it raises problems of informed choice and of the user being able to select safe and efficacious treatments. It is also certainly not the case that older forms of knowledge are 'good' whereas new knowledge is 'bad' or vice versa. This chapter will elaborate on the notion that knowledge is, in fact, ever-changing, subject to fads and fashions and, most of all, affected by power relationships. That is to say, knowledge is neither neutral nor fixed. Those who work with accepted knowledge today might be denounced as quacks or frauds by new knowledge tomorrow. At the same time, there are people whose outright deception and wish to deceive mean the label of 'fraudster' is justified.

This chapter begins by discussing the nature of knowledge and the relationship between the concepts of power and knowledge. Social scientists have been interested in the way forms of knowledge arise and can then maintain power in particular settings (Foucault, 1980; Mennell and Goudsblom, 1988; Delanty, 2000). Some high-status knowledge is culturally valued more than other forms. Here, the focus is on scientific knowledge and how its position as the premier form of knowledge is maintained in contemporary society. It is important to think about science as a form of knowledge because many critiques of CAM stem from the view that it is 'unscientific'. And yet the history of much science can be considered 'unscientific' (Dobraszczyc, 1989). To understand this fully it is necessary to ask questions, such as how did science develop and progress? Also, are there other 'sciences' or approaches to explaining the world that, for one reason or another, cannot challenge orthodoxy? Established forms of knowledge can often be defended and used to attack other forms and it is interesting to identify how they are able to do this.

This chapter goes on to give some examples of disputes **between** different forms of knowledge and **within** forms of knowledge but between factions. Such disputes highlight the political nature of knowledge and often revolve around notions of **authenticity** – who may call themselves a practitioner, the correct forms of training and whether one approach to health and wellbeing is better than another (Gamarnikow, 1978). Also the name-calling and counterclaims of fraud-busting groups are outlined. In these cases, CAM knowledge can be seen as being attacked from outside, by those who claim to represent science and to protect the public. Such claims are sometimes said to be driven by concerns other than the lack of a scientific approach by CAM modalities.

Finally, this chapter looks at how knowledge and expertise about health and wellbeing are accepted by the lay public. In particular, it outlines the social expectations and social conditions that make people place their trust in an astonishing array of forms of health knowledge (both orthodox and CAM).

1.2 Knowledge, value, monopoly and diversity

Different forms of knowledge have varying levels of value in society. Some are more likely to be accepted and believed and have more influence over people's lives. This ranking of information could be termed 'a hierarchy of knowledge', although always bear in mind that this hierarchy is fluid and changeable. Ranking will differ both among cultures and within different sectors of cultures. Individuals may have vastly different personal rankings of the importance of forms of information from each other.

ACTIVITY   DESCRIBING THE WORD 'KNOWLEDGE'

Allow 5 minutes

Look at the definition of knowledge below. It is taken from the Oxford Dictionary and is similar to definitions given in other dictionaries. Given the discussion above about knowledge, power and authority, do you notice anything about this definition and, in particular, how the word 'knowledge' is described?

> **knowledge** familiarity gained by experience (of person, fact or thing); person's range of information (it came to my ~, became known to me; to my ~, so far as I know, as I know for certain); theoretical or practical understanding (of language, subject); some of what is known (every branch of knowledge); **~able** well informed, intelligent.

Comment

You might have noticed that there is no mention of different forms of knowledge having more or less value than others within society. So, the knowledge gained by personal experience is cited as knowledge along with theoretical understanding. This type of description of knowledge has a neutral focus. However, several academic disciplines – such as philosophy, sociology, political theory and social policy – take a very different view of knowledge. These disciplines tend to emphasise the hierarchies of knowledge that define some people as more 'knowledgeable' and have also focused on the way in which knowledge develops, changes and is re-evaluated in different cultural and historical contexts. Furthermore, what might be termed 'high-status knowledge' is always bound up with interest groups and power. For instance, many powerful forms of knowledge in western society are linked to particular occupational or professional groups, leading some commentators to argue that knowledge and power are intimately related (Foucault, 1980).

One of the most interesting facts about knowledge is that it is not contained solely in books or in the minds of people who are considered intellectual or professional. Knowledge is essentially everywhere (see Box 1.1).

BOX 1.1   WHAT IS KNOWLEDGE?

It is easy to think of knowledge as being held or used by people in the professions. However, everyone uses what can be termed 'lay knowledge'. Over time and with experience, individuals gather together ideas, skills, understandings and explanations that help them to go about their lives and deal with the issues at hand. Such knowledge is based on experience with a mixture of knowledge from a range of sources. Groups of ideas and understandings also come together to form sets or groups of knowledge and so it is possible to speak of medical knowledge, osteopathic knowledge, the lay person's knowledge, etc. Such sets of knowledge may disagree with or contradict one another. It can also be said that some forms of knowledge, for whatever reason, are more valued in society than others.

While knowledge can be described as ranked in terms of its importance in society, there is increasing recognition that the knowledge of lay people can positively add to health care provision and practice. For instance, in the case of people with chronic illnesses, such as Parkinson's disease, lay knowledge of how to cope with illness, which home remedies help alleviate symptoms, or practical tips on travelling are very important to the person with the illness. In many cases the medical knowledge of Parkinson's disease cannot answer the day-to-day issues that arise, whereas lay experience and knowledge sometimes can (Pinder, 1988). The importance of harnessing lay information about illness is being recognised by the current government through the expert patient programme (Department of Health, 1999, 2000), in which people with chronic illnesses help others by passing on their lay knowledge.

Box 1.1 shows how health policy is changing towards integrating lay knowledge in some areas. However, such a view obscures the reality that some forms of knowledge are more readily accepted in formal or legal settings as 'real' than others. Thus the patient's view of their illness in the orthodox medical system is usually not valued as much as their consultant's view. The hierarchy of knowledge – or the value placed on one type of knowledge or another – is best seen on those occasions when lay knowledge challenges more formalised and institutionalised knowledge. It is interesting to note how higher-status knowledge can critique other forms of knowledge in these situations. The case study of Camelford illustrates this well.

THE CAMELFORD WATER POISONING: AN EXAMPLE OF LAY AND SCIENTIFIC KNOWLEDGE CLASHING

Water is always a problem in Cornwall: there is usually too little of it during hot summers and too much of it in winter. However, on 6 July 1988, a very different problem arose when a lorry driver accidentally tipped 20 tons of aluminium sulphate solution into the water treatment plant supplying Camelford and the immediate area of North Cornwall. Unfortunately, the accident went undiscovered for some time and local residents and tourists had already drunk the water and began to report side effects. These included vomiting, rashes, nausea, headaches and stomach upsets. Williams and Popay (1994) studied the Camelford poisoning and note that the people affected demanded information from local health professionals, the health authority and the council. The local people also organised to pull together both support and specific expertise within the community. One of the groups formed – Camelford Scientific Advisory Panel (CSAP) – comprised local people with expertise in health and allied areas who monitored people's reports of illness and collated their accounts.

A government committee was given the task of investigating and responding to concerns about the incident (Williams and Popay, 1994). This committee reviewed all the evidence, including that given by the CSAP and the district health authority, and concluded that:

- there had been immediate health effects, experienced by a number of people consuming the water
- the chemicals involved were unlikely to cause problems after such a short term of exposure
- the 'very real health complaints' still visible in the community were probably caused by 'the sustained anxiety naturally felt by many people'.

The report did little to allay public fears about the long-term effects of ingesting the water and the symptoms that many people felt they continued to experience. There was a campaign demanding that the local people's experiences be taken into account properly and, eventually, the governmental committee was reconvened. However, as Williams and Popay note, no local people, other than general practitioners, gave evidence. The second report did not find anything to discount or discredit the first report and there is still public concern about the incident.

Williams and Popay argue that the Camelford incident demonstrates how lay information is often presented as unscientific. In this case, the evidence of lay people was presented as being negatively affected by subjective feelings and emotions. The considerable amount of information accrued by the CSAP and the accounts of illness from local people were discounted as examples of fears and worries. Such thinking and personal experience are seen as unreliable and not as authoritative as scientific and 'objective' information. Yet the knowledge generated by the scientific experts in this case could hardly be said to be neutral. The recent privatisation of the water industry meant that there were good reasons for appointing 'experts' to the committee who held particular views on the effects of ingesting the chemicals (that is, it was relatively safe). There was also the issue of the difficulty of knowing with any certainty the possible long-term effects of drinking water contaminated with aluminium sulphate. The two sides were able to employ scientific 'experts' who had completely different views on this question. This diversity of opinion demonstrates how there is often considerable uncertainty within science, uncertainty that can be used by people with particular agendas. In the Camelford case, lay and local knowledge were written off as less important, despite the fact that it was lay people and local health practitioners who had to deal with the aftermath of the poisoning.

The relative value of different forms of knowledge

There are many other instances that seem to demonstrate the way in which lay knowledge is often seen as secondary or lesser to other forms, for example the debate over the MMR (measles, mumps and rubella) inoculation. These debates have become infused with claims that lay people's fears are subjective or emotionally driven. This is particularly the case in the experience and knowledge of parents who allege their children have suffered because of MMR. Again, as with Camelford, lay people (parents) have often gathered information from other parents about the possible effects of MMR. In the case of the dangers to health from bovine spongiform encephalopathy or BSE (in particular, the risk of acquiring Creutzfeldt-Jakob disease or CJD from meat or blood products), lay people's experiential knowledge was again challenged for some time before scientific research indicated that there was a problem with BSE in humans.

These kinds of examples highlight several issues that need to be taken into account whenever there is a discussion of the relative cultural value placed on different forms of knowledge. These include the way in which some sets of knowledge seem able to claim to be more truthful, scientific, rational and neutral (Latour and Woolgar, 1986); and, alongside this, the way the claims of some sets of knowledge are more likely to be believed and accepted. At the same time, these powerful and authoritative forms of knowledge can discredit others as being less truthful, ill informed or just downright wrong. This process of grading information is a feature of everybody's lives. Ranking information is a necessity in processing it and, although this may well not be a conscious procedure, an important part of this ranking concerns the perceived authority of the person or organisation disseminating the information.

ACTIVITY   WHOSE KNOWLEDGE DO YOU VALUE THE MOST?

Allow 20 minutes

Look at the list below and try to rank who you would value the most to provide information about a sore knee that developed when you got up from kneeling on the floor one day.

- Your local general practitioner (GP)
- A woman who works in the health food shop
- A man who recently had a knee operation
- An osteopath
- A trained physiotherapist (now retired) who lives in your road
- A partner or family friend
- A chiropractor
- A new internet site which provides health information
- A physiotherapist who works privately in your area
- Your local pharmacist
- A massage therapist who you have used for other aches and pains
- NHS Direct – the telephone health helpline run by the National Health Service

After ranking them, look at the top two and the bottom two in your ranking. Does one key factor seem to dominate your choices? What training or knowledge would you prefer people had before giving you advice on this minor health problem?

Comment

You may have found it very difficult to rank these people. Your mind may have been full of 'but what ifs' about particular individuals. To some extent your final choice will be linked to your own experience and beliefs. For some people the GP is the first person they contact, whereas if you use a particular CAM therapy regularly you may have gone for a CAM option. However, if the story of your knee injury were slightly altered – you got up and your knee completely locked or swelled up – your choice of advice-giver might change. This demonstrates that, while there are hierarchies of knowledge and different values placed socially on particular forms of knowledge, individuals may also rank knowledge according to experience, personal preference and the type of problem faced. If, for instance, you believe that your ills are primarily caused by energy imbalances in an aura that exists around your body, you may be more likely to respond to the problem by deciding to visit a CAM practitioner who works with energies. Thus, while there is a hierarchy in society that gives some forms of knowledge a higher cultural status, individuals may also have their own ranking system that may or may not use widespread cultural ideals as a reference point.

Features of high-status knowledge

The key features of high-status knowledge in western society include the following.

- **A privileged status in explaining the world** – the theories offered by this knowledge have more credibility and general acceptance than others at being able to explain phenomena. In other words, this knowledge has an epistemologically privileged position (Latour, 1987).
- **A codified and formalised format** – high-status knowledge is usually written up in texts that map out its basic precepts and thus allow the knowledge to be taught and studied (Faulkner, 1998).
- **Institutionalised and supported knowledge** – high-status knowledge tends to be embodied not only in texts but also in organisations and social structures. Thus medical knowledge is visible everywhere from the physical buildings of hospitals to the social status of being a medical doctor and the power of the British Medical Association.
- **Powerful knowledge** often has the blessing of other powerful institutions, such as the state, and those that have it and use it can exercise considerable authority over others – just because they have this knowledge. It seems to be able to provide information on topics that broadly affect everyone or, at the very least, relates to principles that concern everyone.

■ **Monopoly** – high-status knowledge is also often linked to the concept of monopoly in two ways. First, there is the issue of monopoly over explanation and, second, there is very careful management of who can and cannot have access to that knowledge by those already 'in the know'. Training in 'the knowledge' tends to be closed or guarded, so that those who do train form what sociologists would see as a knowledge elite.

As noted in Box 1.2, powerful knowledge can often be seen as more rational than other forms. Scholars working within the sociology of knowledge have pointed out that the power of particular forms of knowledge is often not about a 'real' ability to describe reality in a true way but more about the creation and maintenance of a set of rules by which reality may be perceived (Latour and Woolgar, 1986; Bloor, 1991). That is to say, forms of knowledge see, describe, explain and interpret the world in a particular way but this way is always open to change.

BOX 1.2   WHAT IS POWER?

Power can be defined as the ability of an individual or a group to make others do their will, even if they do not want to. Authority can be seen as a particular type of power, especially power that is backed by an institutionalised sanction (Mann, 1983, p. 300). Powerful and authoritative knowledge can therefore be seen as sets of information that can make claims that are accepted in society with little resistance. The social scientist Max Weber (1864–1920) argued that, in modern societies, power and authority are often bound up with being able to argue that our knowledge is 'rational' (Weber, 1947; Gerth and Mills, 1948). Groups who claim that their knowledge is based on rational principles can present their ideas as being more authoritative than other groups' ideas.

This was the case during industrialisation and even into the mid-20th century. More recently, however, there seems to have been a move towards a lay rejection of rational authority. Rational knowledge such as science is up against a re-emergence of beliefs in angels, luck, fate and horoscopes, unseen 'subtle' healing energies and unidentified flying objects or UFOs. These ideas seem to challenge rational principles. Even if we accept that the majority of people do not have such beliefs, there seems to be widespread public scepticism in several areas – science, the law, politics, etc. This sometimes leads to 'rational' knowledge being challenged by other people but, as in the case of Camelford, such challenges are not always entirely successful.

This rather difficult idea can be illustrated by the example of a chiropractor and an orthopaedic surgeon looking at an X-ray of the spine of a person who has uncomplicated or 'simple' lower back pain. A chiropractor and an orthopaedic surgeon confronted by the same X-ray will often see it differently. The chiropractor might detect spinal 'lesions' that can be treated through chiropractic treatment. A surgeon looking at the same X-ray may say there is nothing wrong or that some surgical intervention may be necessary. While they are both looking at the same X-ray, they are doing so through differently trained eyes (that is, through their knowledge base). This raises some important questions, such as is knowledge ever really 'true' or certain or accurate and how do established forms of knowledge change and develop over time?

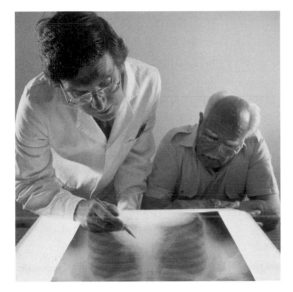

What a health professional and a CAM practitioner see in an X-ray is greatly affected by what they have been trained to look for

Science in perspective

Despite some social antagonism towards it, science is still the justification for much medical dominance. At the same time, it is also the justification for not legitimising other sets of knowledge, such as those propounded by CAM, which have not been or cannot be proven with scientific methods. The idea that knowledge generated by using the scientific method will be neutral and unaffected by the views and opinions of the scientist doing the research is important (Longino, 1990). However, some CAM therapies (especially the Big Five) are developing their authority and credibility by being aligned with an orthodox scientific approach to the knowledge and practice of their modalities (BMA, 2000, p. 9).

The scientific method

The scientific method can be seen as a journey of discovery that takes a scientist from recognising or observing a phenomenon to examining it and being able to verify statements about it, based on research findings. The process often begins with an observation. From this a question is formulated and a hypothesis is developed. For example, a naturalist notices that bees seem to travel around the garden on a certain route. The naturalist develops a hypothesis that this depends on the position of particular plants and that the bees appear to go to the most brightly coloured ones first. Next the naturalist might formulate a prediction that all bees entering the garden will travel in that way, following the brightest flowers. After this the predictions are tested through carefully designed experiments and observations and the data collected are analysed. In particular, the naturalist would take care not to affect the results through their own belief: results should not be affected by the researcher's expectations. When the experiment is finally evaluated there may be one of two outcomes.

1   **The findings support the hypothesis.** The data show that all, or nearly all, bees in the garden follow a path from the brightly coloured flowers to the less bright ones. The naturalist can then decide either to develop this project further in some way or to study another topic.

2   **The findings do not support the hypothesis.** In this case, the naturalist needs to revisit the initial questions, develop them and then go through the scientific method again. The questions may need modification and clarification. If only some of the bees go around the garden in the way initially hypothesised, does the question need modification, such as 'Do the majority of bees from one particular hive follow a route from the most brightly coloured plants to the least bright?'

In this way, the scientific method generates knowledge through neutral observation and experimentation. The results of studies should be replicable, that is they should be repeatable and give the same results for the same or another scientist.

Organised and institutionalised science began around the 17th century but it would be wrong to think that scientific principles, and indeed the scientific method, had not been used to study the world before then. In Ancient Greece, the scientific method was applied to many problems. By the 17th century these ideas were being restored. This was a time of great optimism in scientific principles with a vision that progress could be achieved through a rational and incremental move forward; aspects of the world were to be discovered, tested and mapped by scientific procedures and emerging technologies. The scientific method was the key to developing society. The rapid movement towards accrual of scientific knowledge brought with it confidence that science would (eventually) answer many of the problems that people experience (Latour, 1987).

However, is scientific knowledge always developed through the scientific method? There is a history of theories being discarded because they did not 'fit' with the knowledge of the day and of mistakes in scientific knowledge – blind alleys that did not work out. Medicine did not progress in an even and incremental way. A good example of this is the use of humoral medicine, which was developed in Ancient Greece. It maintained that there were four humors or constituents that made up the body – bile, black bile, blood and phlegm. These constituents had to be in balance for good health and each constituent had certain features that would surface if there was an imbalance. Treatments were designed to redress any imbalances of these constituents of the body. So, if there was too much blood, bloodletting was used. In other cases, emetics (to bring on vomiting) and purgatives (to bring on bowel movements) were prescribed. In the 18th and 19th centuries the notion of the four humors was very much 'in fashion' in medical circles. Indeed, it was a fad that lasted into the 20th century (Dobraszczyc, 1989). At this time, cholera was a massive health problem, killing thousands of people. According to the theory of the four humors, the problem with cholera appeared to be too much moisture in the body. Physicians working within this fashionable medical fad treated patients by bleeding them, sometimes until they were unconscious, and prescribing strong emetics. These treatments had the somewhat unsurprising effect of further weakening the patients and, doubtless, contributed to the number of deaths. However, a study using scientific methods showed that giving people liquids was the best treatment. This research was reported in the medical journal *The Lancet* during the 18th century, but the trends of the day meant it was ignored (Dobraszczyc, 1989). This is a reminder that progress is a difficult concept, beset with allegiances to particular knowledge and techniques.

Surely there is now a different evidence-based attitude to practices? Unfortunately, recent figures on deaths from the 'superbug' MRSA seem to show otherwise. In 2000 approximately 5000 people died from cross-infection in UK hospitals (Kmietowicz, 2000, cited in Elliott, 2003, p. 88). The researchers in this study blamed this shocking figure primarily on a lack of basic handwashing procedures by hospital staff. Hand hygiene is one of the most important barriers against disease transmission, a basic fact that all contemporary health workers are expected to know about and understand. Despite technological progress, fashions, fads and simply ignoring 'evidence' can mean the practices of modern health care are not always backed up by the findings of the scientific method. Another issue is that scientific knowledge emerges that contradicts past advice and confuses the lay public. However, a scientist might argue that there will always be changes in view in science and, as new data emerge, it is only right that the public should be given new advice.

Perhaps one of the main differences between modern medicine and CAM is the ability of the former to define other healing practices in particular ways and its close relationship to more powerful sets of knowledge. Science, and being allied to it, can be a way of justifying knowledge, raising its status and providing a base for claims about the world. For some CAM modalities, science seems to provide ways and means of testing their efficacy and this is actively embraced. For instance, in the case of osteopathy and chiropractic, the scientific knowledge base is growing all the time. Practitioners of these modalities are taught research methods in their training and are expected to produce a piece of research as part of their studies. In the Big Five CAM therapies, although there is still a problem with the number of practitioners having enough research skills and gaining research funding, in general there is no antagonism towards scientific principles and methods. However, across CAM as a whole, the idea of what constitutes 'research' varies tremendously. While it is common for some practitioners to maintain, for instance, that energy has been 'scientifically proven' to exist around the human body, evidence in terms of careful use of the scientific method does not, as yet, exist.

While it is relatively easy to be critical about the scientific method, it provides some checks and measures that can help to protect members of the public, as shown in Box 1.3.

BOX 1.3   IN DEFENCE OF CONTEMPORARY SCIENCE

Science has brought many benefits that most people have experienced at some time in their lives. However, there are reasons why it is useful to challenge the view that science is just like any other form of knowledge. If the argument that all knowledge is the same and that some forms are just more powerful than others is taken to an extreme then there is no way left to judge any knowledge, its utility or contribution to a society. You might want to consider the following statements in relation to whether some level of critical judgement needs to be applied to knowledge.

- Is it all right for an energy healer to claim that they can heal cancer without any evidence?

- Does it matter whether a Chinese herbal preparation on sale in the UK is shown by scientific tests to cause kidney failure, if that is what people want to buy?

- Is it acceptable for a massage practitioner to 'know intuitively' how to work with clients and accidentally injure someone?

- Should a cranial osteopath treat small babies for colic when evidence shows that they tend to get better without this (costly) intervention?

To hold uncritically the belief that science is the same as any other form of knowledge suggests that one form of knowledge is as good as another. While science and medicine are undoubtedly affected by fads, fashions and the failure to adhere to procedure, without the scientific method and the attempt to test one approach to healing against another, people and practitioners have no way of knowing which treatments heal and which ones harm. However, the label 'scientific' does not necessarily guarantee safety or efficacy. There have been some high-profile cases of so-called scientifically proven treatments being harmful, such as the drug thalidomide. This was prescribed to pregnant women in the 1950s to alleviate nausea but resulted in their children being born without limbs.

1.3   Naming, blaming and claiming

In this section some key disputes about knowledge are discussed. Such disputes can arise within CAM modalities (between particular factions), among CAM modalities (for example, disputes about different forms of healing) or between CAM therapies and orthodox knowledge. In some cases, these disputes are about clearly fraudulent and deeply unprofessional behaviour. This discussion begins by looking at some examples of dangerous practice and the 'fraud-busters' who make it their business to identify and publicise bad practice and fraud in CAM.

It is very difficult to define the concept of fraud in relation to CAM. Many modalities do not have formal evidence to back up claims about what they do, so any claim to promote health may be seen as fraudulent or misleading. There are some groups, discussed below, who would define the vast majority of CAM as fraud. While there are certainly cases of direct attempts to confuse or extract money from the public, many claims about 'quacks' are also made by people with extreme anti-CAM views. It is very difficult to draw boundaries between fraud, bad practice or incompetence and a clash of beliefs about health or illness. Often it comes down to points of view.

ACTIVITY   BAD PRACTICE OR FRAUD?

Allow 25 minutes

Read the following excerpt from a newspaper article written by Lucy Atkins (2003). Make notes on the way in which Stephen Hall and Isabella Denley are presented in these accounts.

WHEN THERE'S NO REAL ALTERNATIVE

When Stephen Hall, 43, was diagnosed with inoperable pancreatic cancer, he did what many of us might and went to an alternative therapist who promised him that his condition was curable. Hall believed him. Last week, his 'wellness practitioner', Reginald Gill, 68, from Poole, Dorset, was convicted of two offences under the Trades Descriptions Act after selling Hall an 'IFAS high frequency therapy device' that would, he claimed, kill off the cancer cells. Gill had also advised Hall against chemotherapy, saying he would 'go home in a box' if he did, and told him to stop taking morphine for the pain.

Instead, he put him on an extreme diet, sold him an electronic device, and charged him £75 for treatment sessions at home. The court heard that Gill told Hall after one treatment: 'I've got it. I've killed the bad cells; it's just the pancreas that needs more work.'

Hall died 10 weeks after the cancer was diagnosed. Last week, his mother said outside the court: 'The verdict today should go a long way towards protecting the sick and the terminally ill who, in good faith, go to bogus practitioners who make false claims …' Gill will be sentenced in January.

Clearly, the promises of complementary and alternative medicines (CAMs) can be immensely seductive. About one in five of us use them regularly and millions swear that some therapies cure anything from stress to cancer. But when good sense is replaced by blind faith and mistrust in conventional medicine, the use of CAMs can backfire.

Last year in Melbourne, Australia, Isabella Denley, an epileptic toddler, died after her parents ditched the anti-convulsant medication she had been prescribed by her neurologist. The drugs had terrible side effects, including sleep loss and hyperactivity, so they turned to alternative therapies, visiting a vibrational kinesiologist, a cranial osteopath and a psychic who told them Isabella was suffering from a past-life trauma.

An inquest heard that when she died, the toddler was exclusively on homeopathic medication. Her parents believed they were doing their utmost. But clearly the potential pitfalls of CAMs go beyond ruthless charlatans. Indeed, the real peril may be our faith that alternative therapies will inevitably reach – and cure – the parts that allopathic medicines will not.

'There is certainly evidence to show that some therapies are effective for certain conditions,' says a spokesperson for the Research Council for Complementary Medicine (RCCM). But finding out which ones work for which conditions can be confusing. Often several studies of the same therapy will contradict each other, and since funding for research is hard to come by many studies are considered flawed.

(Source: Atkins, 2003)

Comment

Stephen is portrayed as having somehow lost his way from 'good sense'. Isabella is portrayed more as a victim and her parents as desperate to do the right thing for her. The accounts highlight the negative effects that CAM may have. Words such as 'bogus' and 'charlatan' demonstrate that Atkins feels the people involved in these cases were fraudulent practitioners. However, her article also points the finger at 'non-conventional' medicine in general. The media like nothing better than to find and focus on extreme or unusual examples within CAM or, at the other extreme, to convince people of the benefits of the latest therapy that celebrities are using.

The difficulties of identifying quacks and frauds

There are several words to describe people who mislead others or act in a fraudulent manner about health. The word 'quack' comes from the Old Dutch term 'quacksalver', literally 'to quack like a duck'. It was first used in the 16th century to describe practitioners who boasted about their wares (Gevitz, 1990, p. 2). Interestingly, this definition says nothing about fraud but is mainly about making loud claims and self-advertising. This is probably because, at this time, any person could practise medicine and the notion of 'qualifications' in medicine or health care was meaningless. The doctors of the time had little to offer in terms of skills or remedies and most people could not afford their services. 'Quack' was initially used for both medical and other people. As time went on, and medicine became better organised and more powerful, 'quack' became a more venomous term of abuse that is applied mainly to people who practise outside orthodox medicine. It implies not only boastfulness but also incompetence, whereas 'fraud' is a term used more about the notion of deception and, in particular, the purposeful deception of another person.

Several organisations in the USA are dedicated to monitoring individuals and groups who use forms of knowledge that have little or no evidence base. They include Quackwatch, CSICOP (Committee for the Scientific Investigation of Claims of the Paranormal) and the National Council Against Health Fraud (NCAHF). There are no such organisations in the UK yet, but there are individuals who regularly comment on the fraudulence of CAM, such as James Randi.

Although it is important to detect fraud, it is also necessary to examine those organisations or individuals whose sole purpose is 'fraud-busting' all CAM modalities. However, some difficult issues need unravelling here about what fraud actually is and what factors are used in its definition, including the following.

- The issue of fraud is sometimes mixed up with the issue of efficacy (whether a treatment works or not). If people using CAM say they find particular modalities helpful, but no research has been done to demonstrate this, is it right to label that activity fraudulent? Without evidence there is no way of knowing whether fraud – in the sense of deception – is involved.
- The label 'fraud' may be about entrenched beliefs that either sceptics or CAM advocates hold. These extreme views probably make it difficult for such individuals to accept findings either for or against the usefulness of CAM. For example, in the case of hard-line sceptics, research showing that a CAM therapy does work is likely to be interpreted as fraudulent. As they already believe that CAM is scientifically implausible, they are more likely to argue that there is something wrong with the study involved or the individuals carrying it out or the research conditions, etc.
- Claims of fraud are not limited to groups of sceptics commenting on CAM. Practitioners of CAM are often concerned about other practitioners' competence or use of a style of treatment different from their own.
- Fraud is not the preserve of CAM: there are numerous infamous examples of it in medicine and science.

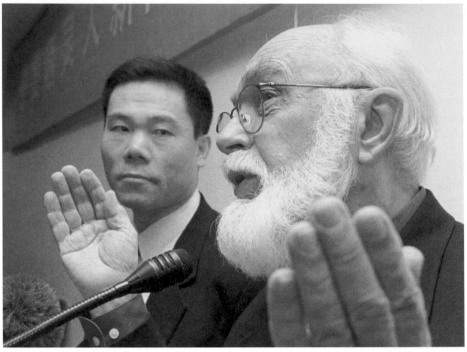

James Randi is one of the most vocal sceptics about CAM. A member of CSICOP, Randi has offered $1 million to anyone who can prove with scientific methods that 'unscientific' phenomena, including many CAM therapies, actually work

These kinds of factors indicate that the label 'fraud' is often intermingled with other disputes over what constitutes acceptable knowledge. Stephen Barrett, a key figure in the US group Quackwatch, argues:

> quackery could be broadly defined as 'anything involving overpromotion in the field of health.' This definition would include questionable ideas as well as questionable products and services, regardless of the sincerity of their promoters. In line with this definition, the word 'fraud' would be reserved only for situations in which deliberate deception is involved. Unproven methods are not necessarily quackery. Those consistent with established scientific concepts may be considered experimental.
>
> (Barrett, 2004)

The central issue for Barrett is that lack of consistency with scientific principles and convention is a defining issue in the label 'quack'. Fraud, however, is 'reserved' for intentional deception.

Knowledge battles within CAM

While CAM practitioners have had to deal with criticism of their knowledge and practice from outside, they have also had to deal with it from within.

There have been knowledge disputes both among CAM modalities and between different factions within them. Many internal disputes have been about personality but also about the knowledge base: that is, what each CAM therapy is about, how it should be taught, who is allowed to call themselves a therapist, etc. As a professional group develops there is a tendency for some people to be excluded and often 'occupational closure' is applied to their ranks (Witz, 1992). This means the professional group takes control of who can and cannot practise, thus placing themselves in a powerful position. Other groups or individuals who could be a threat may be represented in a negative way. A good example of these processes is the way in which formal nursing tried to represent informal women nurses in the 19th century. While the organised nursing set up by Florence Nightingale and others was presented as a pure form of vocation, in which women devoted their lives to the good of others, informal nurses were berated in the press as untrustworthy. Nightingale encouraged the representation of such women as drunks, with little interest in their charges (Gamarnikow, 1978). The point of contention here was authenticity – who was to be allowed to be seen as a 'real' nurse and who was not? It was in the professional self-interest of nursing to develop control over who could and could not be allowed to practise. As Mary Chamberlain notes: 'Medicine, like war, is an extension of politics ... A story of control and access' (1981, p. 139). In the same way, disputes within CAM modalities and among different ones are often about authenticity and control.

Disputes over authenticity, practice, qualifications and name

Naturopathy or 'nature cure' is a form of therapy that uses natural methods to help the body regain health. One of the key ideas of this modality is that 'only nature heals' (Power, 1994, p. 195). Natural methods for helping the body attain health include reviewing and then increasing the nutritional quality of the diet, fresh air, sunshine and exercise. The therapy aims to help the user through minimum intervention. Naturopathy is a good example of knowledge differences within a CAM. These differences revolve around which methods are natural and which are not, and can affect whether a practitioner joins a particular naturopathic professional organisation and how they are viewed by their colleagues. Power (1994) notes that there are differences of opinion about what minimum intervention is. For some, who are often referred to in naturopathy as 'straight nature cure practitioners' (Power, 1994), anything that could be construed as a remedy is not acceptable. However, some naturopaths now favour the use of nutritional supplements to aid the diet of users. They argue that modern foods have less nutritional value and therefore supplementation is needed now in a way that it was not in the past. Such an approach is vehemently opposed by others who see it as a move away from the traditional approach of naturopathy.

The dispute is about the essential knowledge base of naturopathy and whether or not the modality should change in the face of contemporary life.

Disputes arise in other modalities, not only about the authenticity of practitioners (who the real practitioners are) but also about how the principles of a modality may be interpreted in the context of the western world. Many CAM therapies which originated in the East are now practised in the West, giving rise to concerns about whether aspects of traditional practice have been lost. Reiki is a form of energy-based healing from Japan. Developed in the late 18th and early 19th centuries by Dr Usui, it is allegedly based on much older Buddhist principles. Practitioners believe that they can channel universal energy through their hands and into another person. This ability is passed to a student by a Master through a process called **attunement**. This involves passing down from Master to student oral history and a set of rituals in which the healing ability is passed on. Once a person is 'attuned', they are said to have joined their Master's 'lineage'. Similar to a family tree, people who have been attuned can be traced back through their Masters in a chain of training. Although there was once only one form of reiki – that developed by Usui – other forms have emerged and there are now over 20 different ones in the UK. As in all CAM therapies, there has been internal disagreement about reiki. In particular, there are concerns about how the knowledge about reiki should be passed on. In early reiki training in Japan a student studied for about a year to gain a first degree (the initial training) and another year or more for a second degree. A first degree in the UK now more usually takes about two days but other courses combine both first and second degrees in two days. Some practitioners believe that such shortened training is dangerous and also inauthentic to the traditions of reiki, as explained by Peter Warnock, a reiki Master. He argues that students do not have 'the necessary integration period between the degrees which energetically has the effect of reversing the first degree attunement, stunting the individual's personal healing process and placing unnecessary strain on their energy fields' (Warnock, 2000, p. 3).

Warnock also points out his concerns about the central precepts and values of reiki and whether they are being honoured. This has been a concern for many practitioners after attempts worldwide to patent reiki healing by particular groups or Masters. Patenting would lead to one person or group having the power to define who could or could not use the name 'reiki'. This led Phyllis Furomoto, who sits at the top of the worldwide lineage of reiki, to try to patent reiki in the USA and other countries. Her argument for doing this was to block the way of those who would patent reiki and then use it in an exclusionary manner. In gaining the patent, Furomoto said she would allow reiki to continue as it was – open to all. Other divisions in the reiki community have been created by some practitioners publishing sacred symbols – which some argue should be taught only by Masters – in books or on the internet (for example, Stein, 1995). There are more general disputes among practitioners about particular types of reiki being more 'powerful' than others. Reiki does not yet have an overarching regulatory body in the UK, although currently there is a working group that involves the majority (but not all) of reiki professional groups. However, disputes that focus on how reiki should be practised and the basic philosophical approach to teachings make integration very difficult.

Sometimes disputes arise within a CAM modality when it is going through formal professionalisation processes, such as developing statutory self-regulation (SSR). In these cases, strict new rules and the expectations of practitioners can lead to the exclusion of some individuals. An example of this is what happened to some people practising under the name of 'osteopath' when the Osteopaths Act 1993 was passed and a central register of practitioners set up. At this time a new term arose in the CAM vocabulary – 'osteomyologist'. While it is true that this term is used now by people who were not practising under the title 'osteopath' at this time, it initially emerged as a title used by people who were either excluded or disillusioned by the move to regulation under the Act.

The changes embodied by the Act meant that only members of the General Osteopathic Council (GOC), who paid yearly subscriptions and submitted to rules such as undertaking continuing professional development, could use the title 'osteopath'. The changes did allow for those who had worked as osteopaths for some years, but who had no formal training, to gain entrance to the register by submitting a portfolio of work. This allowance is termed a 'grandfather clause' and is often used when groups professionalise. However, some practitioners viewed submitting this work as belittling and/or they found creating the portfolio difficult. Furthermore, the fees expected by the GOC were prohibitive for some practitioners, thus providing a further disincentive for registration. For a small minority, their submitted portfolios were not of acceptable quality. While the move to SSR was heralded as a success by the GOC, clearly some practitioners lost out in this process and could no longer practise under the title 'osteopath'. Currently, osteopaths trained in accredited GOC educational institutions automatically gain the right to register on graduation. Chapter 3 deals specifically with the issue of regulation.

These cases demonstrate the political and contentious nature of knowledge within CAM. In the case of the meaning of 'nature cure', there is a dispute over what constitutes authentic naturopathic practice. In reiki there are issues of both authenticity and ownership of the modality and its knowledge. Lastly, the case of the osteomyologists shows that regulation can lead to bitter disputes as some practitioners become defined as not having the correct knowledge to practise under a particular title. Knowledge disputes within CAM can be as bitter and sometimes intractable as those between CAM and other forms of knowledge.

1.4 Trust, knowledge and expectations: CAM users and deception

When knowledge is described as having some power or widespread authority, it is also necessary to speak of trust. The creation of trusting therapeutic relationships is at the core of successful CAM practice. Trust can be seen as operating within situations 'in which an individual's ability to assess risk or probability is absent and yet they still choose to believe something' (Lee-Treweek, 2003, p. 49).

With so many different sets of knowledge available, people can trust a treatment or therapist who does not deserve it. Although some of the fraud-busters who seek to demonstrate that CAM involves deception appear to have extreme views, every year people are deceived by practitioners who make false claims. Although some forms of knowledge have authority in society, others may become important to people regardless of whether they have the backing of society in general. For example, some people visit reiki healers or spiritual surgeons even though these forms of healing are not legitimated by mainstream culture. This naturally leads to the question of why people choose to place their trust in particular CAM practices or individuals.

Having a sense of trust in a CAM therapy or therapist involves several factors that can be split into macro (or large-scale) issues and micro (small-scale interaction or communication) issues. Macro issues include:

■ whether the knowledge is well known and (allegedly) backed up by a dominant and authoritative knowledge such as science
■ whether the knowledge is institutionalised and generally accepted, such as knowledge that is institutionalised into the National Health Service
■ whether there is suddenly a fashion or fad in society for particular CAM therapies, which may be legitimated by celebrity or royal usage, widespread coverage on television, and so on.

Although these macro factors are very important, what actually happens between a practitioner and a user is of key importance to the development of trust.

Micro issues include:

■ an individual's expectations of the therapy or practitioner
■ whether the practitioner is interpreted as honest, competent, etc.
■ whether the user feels a sense of connection to the practitioner.

Personal judgements and expectations may be more important in deciding to trust a practitioner than checking credentials or qualifications (Lee-Treweek, 2003). Given that personal evaluations are important in building up trust, it is easy to see that users could be deceived by a practitioner who is fraudulent or just misguided.

So, building trust between user and practitioner relies on personal interpretations. Users of CAM are likely to choose particular practitioners because there is a perception of personal liking or connection. This is similar, of course, to people's choice of many other health professionals. This sense of connection may relate to the user's feeling of congruence with the ideas of health that the practitioner holds and/or a personal assessment of their character and personality. There have been some recent high-profile cases of orthodox health-care practitioners who convinced people around them that they were trustworthy, when clearly they were not. For example, paediatric nurse Beverley Allitt and the disgraced GP Harold Shipman used their positions to injure and murder people in their care, while at the same time appearing to colleagues and families to be a competent and caring person (Horton, 2001). It seems that user perception combined with expectation is important in choosing to trust. People who want to deceive or create a false sense of being trustworthy, whether in CAM or orthodox health work, can manipulate these factors to their own ends.

1.5   Conclusion

This chapter has discussed the way in which some knowledge forms are high status and how knowledge is ranked in society. Such ranking will vary both among societies and among different individuals who may not use societal values as a reference point for their own beliefs. The resurgence of CAM since the 1960s illustrates the growing number of people who no longer place their full trust in conventional forms of science or orthodox medicine. It would be easy to say disputes over knowledge are the preserve of science versus other sets of knowledge, but this is not the case. There are hotly contested debates within CAM about the nature of therapies, what constitutes an authentic practitioner and what is accepted as evidence of efficacy. While some CAM therapists seem to hold views that are completely antithetical to conventional science, others acknowledge that science is a possible way of justifying CAM therapies and beliefs, and yet others embrace scientific methods completely.

There are considerable problems in defining what fraudulent practice in CAM is today. The vulnerability of the public or safety issues are often cited as the justification for labelling some therapists as fraudsters, and clearly there are incompetent and dangerous practitioners or those who use CAM as a vehicle to deceive other people for financial gain. Those who do use overt deception have a wide range of expectations and beliefs that can help them dupe the public. However, other claims of fraud seem based on the values of those making the claim. This is particularly the case in disputes within CAM modalities about the authenticity of specific groups of practitioners. There is also a tension between rooting out deception on the one hand and, on the other, seeing CAM as operating in an open marketplace in which people are free to believe in anything that makes their life more meaningful. Understanding how people trust others seems to suggest that preventing deception in CAM is therefore very difficult.

KEY POINTS

- Sets of knowledge are ranked by both society and individuals – they are culturally accepted and legitimated to different extents.

- Fights between high and low status knowledge show the differences in the way forms of knowledge are valued. In the case of Camelford, lay knowledge was defined as less scientific, more subjective and personal and therefore less likely to be 'true'.

- The notion of objective knowledge obscures the fact that knowledge is not neutral, arises within particular conditions and is contested by other forms of knowledge that may actually supersede it at some point.

- Name-calling and labelling others as frauds or quacks is a common strategy with a long history and is used both within CAM (between different modalities) and against CAM by other bodies (such as fraud-busting organisations). This excludes some CAM practitioners from either using a particular name or being seen as a proper practitioner. These internal disputes have arisen about issues such as the use of particular techniques, what constitutes 'proper' education or training or the philosophical basis of the modality.

- Research on orthodox health care suggests that, despite the rhetoric on the use of evidence, health care is not always based on the latest scientific principles.

- The social expectations of CAM users can contribute towards being deceived or defrauded.

- Generally it is difficult to separate fraudsters or deception from good-willed practitioners because of the nature of CAM knowledge and its (lack of) a scientifically accepted evidence base.

References

Atkins, L. (2003) 'When there's no real alternative', *The Guardian*, 15 December.

Barrett, S. (2004) 'Quackery, how should it be defined?' [online], www.quackwatch.org/01QuackeryRelatedTopics/quackdef.html [accessed 16 January 2004].

Bloor, D. (1991) *Knowledge and Social Imagery* (2nd edition), Chicago, University of Chicago Press.

British Medical Association (BMA) (2000) *Acupuncture: Efficacy, Safety and Practice*, London, Harwood/BMA.

Chamberlain, M. (1981) *Old Wives' Tales*, London, Virago.

Delanty, G. (2000) *Modernity and Postmodernity: Knowledge, Power and the Self*, London, Sage.

Department of Health (1999) *Saving Lives: Our Healthier Nation*, London, HMSO.

Department of Health (2000) *The NHS Plan*, London, HMSO.

Dobraszczyc, U. (1989) *Sickness, Health and Medicine*, Harlow, Longman.

Elliott, P. (2003) 'Recognising the psychosocial issues involved in hand hygiene', *The Journal of the Royal Society for the Promotion of Health*, Vol. 123, No. 2, pp. 88–94.

Faulkner, W. (1998) 'Knowledge flows in innovation', in Williams, R., Faulkner, W. and Fleck, J. (eds) *Exploring Expertise: Issues and Perspectives*, pp. 173–96, London, Macmillan.

Foucault, M. (1980) *Power/Knowledge* (edited by Colin Gordon), Brighton, Harvester Press.

Gamarnikow, E. (1978) 'Sexual division of labour: the case of nursing', in Kuhn, A. and Wolpe, A. M. (eds) *Feminism and Materialism: Women and Modes of Production*, pp. 97–100, 105–107 and 121, London, Routledge.

Gerth, H. and Mills, C. W. (eds) (1948) *Essays from Max Weber*, London, Routledge and Kegan Paul.

Gevitz, N. (1990) 'Three perspectives on unorthodox medicine', in Gevitz, N. (ed.) *Other Healers*, Baltimore, MD, Johns Hopkins University Press.

Horton, C. (2001) 'Safeguards were not tough enough admits DoH', *The Guardian*, 5 January.

Latour, B. (1987) *Science in Action*, Harvard, Harvard University Press.

Latour, B. and Woolgar, S. (1986) *Laboratory Life: The Social Construction of Scientific Facts* (2nd edition), Princeton, NJ, Princeton University Press.

Lee-Treweek, G. (2003) 'Trust in complementary medicine: the case of cranial osteopathy', *The Sociological Review*, Vol. 50, No. 1, pp. 48–68.

Longino, H. (1990) *Science as Social Knowledge*, Princeton, NJ, Princeton University Press.

Mann, M. (1983) *Macmillan Student Encyclopaedia of Sociology*, London, Macmillan.

Mennell, S. and Goudsblom, J. (eds) (1988) *Norbert Elias on Civilization, Power and Knowledge: Selected Writings*, Chicago, University of Chicago Press.

Pinder, R. (1988) 'Striking a balance: living with Parkinson's disease', in Anderson, R. and Bury, M. (eds) *Living with Chronic Illness*, London, Unwin Hyman.

Power, R. (1994) 'Only nature heals', in Budd, S. and Sharma, U. (eds) *The Healing Bond*, London, Routledge.

Stein, D. (1995) *Essential Reiki*, Freedom, CA, The Crossing Press.

Warnock, P. (2000) 'The training and practice of Reiki', *The Therapist*, Issue 3, December. Available online at www.iptiuk.com/the_therapist/therapist3.html [accessed 22 December 2004].

Weber, M. (1947) *The Theory of Social and Economic Organisations*, London, Free Press.

Williams, G. and Popay, J. (1994) 'Lay knowledge and the privilege of experience', in Gabe, J., Kellaher, D. and Williams, G. (eds) *Challenging Medicine*, London, Routledge.

Witz, A. (1992) *Professions and Patriarchy*, London, Routledge.

Chapter 2 Education and training in CAM

Lorraine Williams, Julie Stone and Geraldine Lee-Treweek

Contents

AIMS

- To promote knowledge and understanding of the history and evolution of CAM education and training.
- To explore the diversity and variation of education and training both among and within different CAM therapies.
- To discuss the debates and dilemmas in CAM education and training.

2.1 Introduction

Education and training for practitioners of complementary and alternative medicine (CAM) is a major factor in ensuring the quality of service to users and for the status and credibility of the practitioners. Basically, education and training need to provide practitioners with a satisfactory level of knowledge and skills to be safe and competent in their particular modality. This chapter explores the type of education and training suited to CAM, as well as who best provides it. Perhaps more importantly, it addresses the many contentious issues that arise in trying to provide appropriate education and training to the diverse group of modalities that make up CAM. In the UK, CAM modalities have evolved with the comparative freedom of unrestricted practice, which has encouraged creativity and growth. At the same time, however, this has allowed a proliferation of qualifications and practice of varying standards and quality. As CAM becomes increasingly popular with orthodox health care practitioners and within integrated health service settings, the nature and quality of CAM education and training are under increased scrutiny.

In the more established therapies, education and training are increasingly located within the higher and further education (HFE) sectors. Courses within these institutions are required to have the same quality controls as the training of orthodox health professionals, but this is not necessarily the case in the less well established therapies. The House of Lords Select Committee notes 'CAM training courses vary in their content, depth and duration, both between disciplines and in some cases within the same discipline' (2000, para. 6.1). In such a climate, it may be hard for a potential client to know whether the practitioner they consult is competent or not (Stone, 2002).

This chapter begins by exploring the development of CAM education and training from the informal transmission of knowledge into more formal models of provision. Initially the informal route included handing down traditional knowledge through community healers and therapists whose style was charismatic or personality-driven. More recently, private colleges have become important in the development of training and education in CAM and the HFE sectors have become increasingly involved in this provision. However, the suggestion is not that more formal models of training are better or more appropriate. Certainly formal educational approaches (which are increasingly seen as requiring external accreditation) are one of the hallmarks of professionalisation, along with effective regulatory structures. For CAM therapies seeking professional status in the eyes of the government and the general public, the way in which their practitioners are trained is increasingly recognised as an area that requires formal structures. The subject of professionalisation is addressed more fully in Chapter 4.

This chapter concludes by considering some current controversies in CAM education. It asks whether there should be a core curriculum for all CAM modalities; the extent to which CAM education requires training in basic medical sciences – including anatomy and physiology; the need for continuing professional development (CPD); and how knowledge or 'familiarisation' with CAM might best be integrated into the curricula of orthodox health care courses.

2.2 Historical issues of training and education in CAM

Before the rise of biomedicine as the dominant form of health knowledge in western societies there was a plural marketplace: herbalists, healers and psychics coexisted with groups that were the forerunners of the medical profession today – physicians, barber/surgeons and apothecaries (Porter, 1999). The notion of a 'CAM practitioner' only emerged by default as the profession of medicine became increasingly dominant and insisted on demarcating orthodox medicine from other (complementary or alternative) forms of health care practice. Attempts to professionalise orthodox medical practice through the foundation of the Royal College of Physicians in the 16th century marked the first level of separation between orthodox medical practice and CAM. However, 'complementary' practice still flourished in the 16th, 17th and 18th centuries because most people could not afford the luxury of a graduate physician.

Most people's health needs were dealt with at home by family members or by lay people in their local communities (Dobraszczyc, 1989). Mary Chamberlain documents several remedies that were used in the household (1982, p. 42). These involved all manner of unusual ingredients, such as bits of dead insect, willowherb and fresh moss from a churchyard skull. At the same time, other individuals who were considered to be healers within the community – the so-called 'wise women' and 'cunning men' – were skilled in using remedies and making charms and amulets, using prayer and removing curses. Any training would have been entirely informal and based on passing down oral folk knowledge. It is also worth remembering that people calling themselves 'doctors' almost certainly had little more knowledge than lay people of how to deal with illness and disease. Indeed, these different groups often shared therapeutic remedies and were virtually indistinguishable from each other. In the medical marketplace, people who could afford to use university-trained doctors often did so for status reasons, to show they could afford a doctor, rather than for reasons of increased efficacy.

However, even people using the title 'doctor' had training that varied in depth and type. It was not until the mid-19th century that there was a serious attempt to regulate medical practice with the passing of the Medical Registrations Act 1858. A few 'doctors' had degrees from universities such as Oxford, Cambridge and Edinburgh and some trained in Europe. In general, however, successful practice depended on pleasing clients and fashion, in particular being competitive or using flattery (Porter, 1999) – so-called 'bedside medicine' – rather than having clinical skill and competence. Orthodox medical training developed in the 1800s as private schools of anatomy were established. Many hospitals in London were used to develop training in clinical practice for medical students, and partnerships formed between universities and hospitals. During the 1800s several new CAM therapies were 'discovered'. Initially they did not have formal training programmes but the founders passed on the basic concepts to interested people through enthusiastic personality-driven training. The successful future of these new medical approaches rested on whether the founders could attract new 'followers' who wanted to learn more and become practitioners themselves. Sarah Cant (1996) calls this way of recruiting and training people through enthusiasm **charismatic training**. She notes that many CAM therapies move through an early period of charismatic training into more formal phases, which then develop further on the basis of the CAM itself, rather than the personality of the teacher.

ACTIVITY   THE QUALITIES OF GOOD TEACHING

Allow 10 minutes

Drawing on your own experiences of being taught, either at school or later in life, rank the qualities of teaching listed below in terms of their importance to you as a learner. In other words, which qualities of teaching most helped you to learn?

| Enthusiastic | Knowledgeable | Inspirational | Understandable |
| Confident | Scholarly | Methodical | Engaging |

Comment

Clearly, all of these qualities are important. Enthusiasm without knowledge is probably not enough but often the more personal qualities of the teacher create the best atmosphere for learning. If education and training in CAM developed entirely away from more personality-driven forms of training, it could lose some of the more inspired ways of teaching.

Complementary practice grew less popular as the new 'enlightened' biomedical orthodoxy achieved cultural dominance. This was not the case with homeopathy, which retained some popularity during this time, was patronised by royalty (Nicholls, 2005) and often practised by orthodox medical practitioners as well as lay people. The creation of the National Health Service (NHS) in 1948 confirmed biomedicine as the dominant form of health care in the UK. However, lay people still used home remedies and an interest in CAM remained. As Bakx (1991) notes, alternative forms of healing other than biomedicine were 'eclipsed' during this time, rather than being dominated or eradicated. However, in the 1960s there was a resurgence of interest in CAM and training providers began to proliferate. At this time, 'new' CAM therapies began to join those that were indigenous or traditional to the UK (such as certain types of herbalism). In particular, CAM therapies either from or inspired by other cultures became visible in the landscape of health practice, for example reiki, shiatsu and traditional Chinese medicine.

In this developing and diverse CAM landscape, charismatic training did not just disappear. Indeed, Cant (1996) does not suggest that forms of CAM always develop away from charismatic models; many forms of CAM today are still based on the importance of inspirational individuals or charismatic teaching. The following are examples of how personality or charisma still affects training.

- Some training still revolves around the name or personality of one person. Schools or colleges of some modalities are named after one trainer who may teach the whole course. The attraction of such colleges often rests on the characteristics of that individual. In other instances whole techniques in CAM rest on the philosophy of one person, such as Rudolf Steiner's movement-based therapy 'eurhythmy'.
- Other training revolves around the trainee working 'one-to-one' with the CAM trainer using a guru–follower model. For example, reiki training for 'master' level usually involves one-to-one intensive training, along with the supervised treatment of users. In this instance, charismatic training usually involves the trainee and the trainer selecting each other for the connection or congruence they have with each other. In reiki that type of congruent and close training could be considered a strength, not a weakness. Other CAM therapies that may involve this sort of training include some forms of shamanism and healing energy work.

There is nothing inherently wrong with charismatic training and it is wrong to assume that, because some CAM practices evolved or changed from charismatic to formal styles, all of them would follow this route. However, styles of training do have consequences in terms of trying to maintain quality and parity between different training providers or teachers and the variability of student experiences. Setting standards or benchmarking to improve service provision, protection of the public and the creation of consistency are increasingly important in a variety of settings in contemporary society. In CAM education, as in education more generally, setting standards is seen as a key way of raising its profile and status. National Occupational Standards (NOSs) have been developed for several CAM therapies and are being developed for others. The government-funded organisation responsible for them is called Skills for Health. Its task is to produce frameworks that measure the performance of practitioners. Theoretically such frameworks are being developed in collaboration with organisations and stakeholders, thus bringing groups together to develop standards for the skills that could be expected of particular types of practitioner. These NOSs can then be used as a source of information for individuals, professional bodies and education providers and for those responsible for maintaining standards in the workplace (Skills for Health, 2003). However, getting diverse groups to collaborate and take part in consultation exercises is difficult, especially when there are deeply rooted differences within many CAM modalities and between different factions.

2.3 Diversity of training among and within different CAM therapies

As the public popularity of CAM has increased, the HFE and university sectors have become more involved in providing CAM training or working in partnership with private establishments to share provision. In these contexts, additional educational standard frameworks are being applied, such as higher education benchmarks, and courses have to meet standards similar to those for orthodox health care courses.

ACTIVITY   DO EDUCATION AND TRAINING HAVE MIXED MEANINGS?

Allow 20 minutes

The terms 'education' and 'training' are both used in this chapter. However, they can describe different approaches. Explore your understanding of these terms by listing the attributes you can think of under the headings 'education' and 'training'.

Comment

Although the terms 'education' and 'training' may sometimes be used interchangeably, you may have noted down some differences similar to those below.

Education	Training
Broad based	Task or competence orientated
Acquiring knowledge 'of' or knowledge 'about'	Knowledge of 'how to'
Knowledge-driven	Often tailored towards needs of employers
Leads to academic qualification	Prepares individual for professional practice
Does not necessarily anticipate practice	Anticipates employment or practice
Historically, classroom-based	Clinic or work-based
Exam-based assessment	Skills-based assessment

Generally, education suggests something broader that may be longer term. Training implies a focused form of study or learning, usually with a skills-based approach. If these terms are applied to the study of particular CAM therapies, it may be difficult to separate them in practice. For instance, osteopathy involves both skills-based learning in a clinic and more theoretical classroom study of disciplines such as psychology and sociology to understand the broader context of health and illness in society. Students of osteopathy may well be offered a broader education based around the nature of human experience as well as skills-based training. This could be compared and contrasted with a one-day training course in Indian head massage, which focuses on the skills needed to do this but may not provide a good understanding of wider social issues.

Overview of current provision of CAM training

Five different types and levels of courses in complementary health care can be identified, as described below. Courses at the first two levels could be suitable entry routes to practitioner level courses, although not to degree level courses, in some therapies.

1 Self-development or self-help courses

These provide an introduction that is sufficient for the student to apply the therapy in a limited way to themselves, although they are sometimes advertised as enabling the student to apply the therapy to family and friends. They are not practitioner level courses and not all therapies are suitable for such courses. For instance, Bach flower remedies can be successfully self-applied but chiropractic is not appropriate. Some of these courses may be self-study or distance-learning courses.

2 Introductory level courses

These introduce the therapy but do not enable the student to apply or practise it in any way. They are often called introductory or 'taster' courses.

3 Practitioner level courses

These equip the student to practise complementary health care in order to treat the general public. They are commonly referred to as **professional qualifications**. They are often diploma courses but could be degrees or higher national certificates instead. Some may be part of wider qualifications, for instance aromatherapy as part of a degree in health sciences. Others may be a degree or diploma in themselves, such as a BSc in herbal medicine.

4 Academic theory courses

These courses give the student an academic level of knowledge and understanding of complementary health care. They are often aimed at qualified health practitioners (orthodox and complementary) who want to further their general knowledge and understanding of complementary health care. They do not always include professional training but often form part of a degree in health studies and are usually offered through a university. They may also be available as a distance-learning package. Qualified practitioners can use these courses as part of their CPD programme. The courses are also of interest to anyone wanting to gain a general critical awareness of complementary health care but who does not aim to practise the therapy, for instance health care managers, health promoters and environmental health officers.

5 Professional practice and development courses

These courses are aimed at qualified health care practitioners and are often offered as certificates in specialised practice, such as complementary therapies within palliative care or pain control, or as theory-based modules.

Training providers for CAM

CAM is characterised by a diversity of training outlets with a variety of approaches to teaching CAM. The British Medical Association's report (1993), while broadly supporting initiatives and developments in CAM, still had reservations about training, who could train in CAM, the standards of that training, and how the public could be sure they were being treated by a trained, competent person. A key difficulty in the contemporary provision of CAM is the variation in styles of training available.

Private colleges

The teaching of many CAM therapies has developed largely in the private sector. The majority of private colleges offer their own qualification at the end of the course (usually a diploma). Other courses, particularly distance-learning courses, may not lead to an approved practitioner award. Some courses, but by no means all, are validated (recognised and given higher education degree or diploma status) by universities or other national awarding bodies. The following issues should be considered.

- Quality control: there can sometimes be a lack of independent validation of educational standards, including the standard of training, the appropriateness of level and content, and the teaching and learning environment. Some courses are externally validated by HFE institutions, in which case quality is monitored thoroughly.

- They may not have connections or contacts with wider health care stakeholders and professional networks.
- Historically, they are likely to offer graduates entry to their own 'professional' register.
- They may be linked to the provision of goods, products or specific services; for example, training at aromatherapy school may allow only their own registered practitioners to retail certain products.

Colleges of further education

Many colleges of further education offer courses in complementary health care, predominantly in therapies such as aromatherapy, reflexology and massage. Often they offer a nationally recognised qualification, such as a diploma, from an awarding body that is regulated by one of the UK statutory regulating authorities: the Qualifications and Curriculum Authority (QCA) in England, Wales and Northern Ireland and the Scottish Qualifications Authority (SQA) in Scotland. They are also beginning to provide standardised training with curricula linked to NOSs. These standards are discussed in depth in Section 2.5 but, for now, they represent sets of competencies that a range of stakeholders have worked together to identify as standards for the particular modality.

   Some colleges have formed partnerships with local universities and offer foundation degrees in complementary therapies, with therapy pathways leading to practitioner qualifications. Course providers are now seeking accreditation (professional recognition) for many of these courses. Other courses offered in this sector include diplomas in holistic practice, offering more than one therapy (usually a combination of massage, aromatherapy, reflexology, nutrition and counselling skills), with training to practitioner diploma level in each therapy. This kind of cross-specialisation can be very useful for prospective students who want broad-based practitioner training.

Universities

Denise Rankin-Box (2001), a commentator on educational developments in CAM, claims that there are more than 20 universities in the UK offering a range of undergraduate and postgraduate courses and modules in CAM. Even within this sector there is diversity. Some universities offer higher education diplomas, degrees or masters programmes in individual complementary therapies, which would include training to practitioner level as part of the degree or diploma. Many universities offer combined degrees in health studies with complementary medicine as an option, although these are not always to practitioner level. Other degrees in complementary medicine, therapies or health care offer pathways to professional practice, often in aromatherapy or reflexology, although not all have accreditation from the therapy's professional bodies. Many universities offer postgraduate qualifications such as masters programmes aimed at complementary as well as orthodox health care practitioners. All these courses have a high academic content but do not necessarily offer any clinical experience and, therefore, may not develop the skills needed for the competent and safe practice of a particular CAM. University courses, although providing academic qualifications, do not give students of CAM the licence to practise. However, some courses are recognised by particular CAM professional bodies, which accept graduates on to their professional register and so they can get insurance to practise, etc.

With such a range of training on offer, it can be difficult for a prospective student to decide on a course. The case study in Box 2.1 illustrates some of the often bewildering array of choices facing prospective CAM students. It describes how one would-be CAM student reached her decision. Of course, her experiences are not the same for every prospective student in CAM but anyone trying to find the right course for them is likely to encounter similar factors.

BOX 2.1   SUE DECIDES TO TRAIN IN SHIATSU

Sue is a member of the team who developed this book. Recently she began her first year of training in shiatsu, a traditional hands-on Japanese healing art. It allegedly works with the energies of the body, helping to promote the flow of energy and enhancing both health and wellbeing. Sue became increasingly interested in CAM after visiting a shiatsu practitioner and receiving treatment for migraine headaches. Her first experience of treatment had a profound effect on her as she found it relaxing and interesting. After this Sue tried acupuncture and discovered that both shiatsu and acupuncture worked with energy fields believed to be in the body called meridians. While she found both modalities useful for her health, she preferred the closeness between the user and practitioner in shiatsu and found the touch aspect therapeutic. This led her to want to train but she was faced with a large number of training establishments to choose from. How could she decide between them? There were some particular concerns that were important to Sue: first, price was important because she had a fixed budget and travelling far would be difficult, so she needed to find something within a 50-mile radius of home. As a full-time employee and mother, Sue had to take into account the time and scheduling of courses as she had other commitments to fulfil. In order to become a competent practitioner once the course was finished, she accepted that it may take a few years of study given the other constraints in her life. So she decided that a part-time course that was run at the weekends, as close to home as possible and within a £2000 a year budget would be best. Searches on the internet indicated that there were not only a range of providers but also several professional bodies offering training. Sue decided to ask for advice from the practitioner she had used originally. The practitioner suggested a small private school but, unfortunately, the next course was not running for some time. The principal of this course suggested another school and Sue decided to call them and see what they could offer her.

Sue rang the principal of the college recommended by her first choice college. The principal spent a long time discussing the course, its structure and rationale. She was enthusiastic about her modality and also demonstrated awareness of the importance of practitioners' ethical behaviour. Sue particularly liked the fact that the first section of the course was designed as a 'taster' to allow potential students to decide whether they really wanted to invest in the full course. The final issue that enabled Sue to choose this course was that she felt she got on well with the principal and that they shared a similar set of ideas around health and healing. While the depth of the curriculum, geographical proximity and cost were important factors to her, ultimately Sue's decision rested on her sense of trust in the person who designed and ran the course.

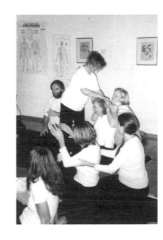

Students being trained at the Genki School of Shiatsu

Is the proliferation of education and training in CAM 'a good thing'?

The diversity of providers of CAM education and training and the range of qualifications on offer mean that potential students often have little knowledge of whether the training they have chosen is of a high standard and/or will provide the skills they need to become competent practitioners. However, there are some 'gold standards' that denote some forms of training as being more rigorous than others – notably, externally validated and accredited courses. External validation involves a course being endorsed and often certified by an external body in order to meet stringent quality criteria. This type of course is established as the preferred model in orthodox health care education. Many private colleges validate their own courses or may have some input from one of the many professional bodies in their field. Some private colleges also accredit their own courses, which means the qualification attained at the end of the course is not recognised anywhere except by the college itself. In this situation it is hard for potential students to judge how their training will be viewed by orthodox health care professionals, other practitioners in the modality, and so on. Furthermore, claims made in advertising materials about the college having good standards or being validated by a particular body can create a false sense of the importance or significance of the training they provide. Often there are also claims of being more 'authentic' than other colleges, or that one college teaches methods that other colleges do not offer. Such claims draw attention to the nature of training as an entrepreneurial as well as a teaching endeavour. It also goes against the concept of good practice put forward in the House of Lords report:

> We recommend that CAM training courses should become more standardised and be accredited and validated by the appropriate professional bodies. All those who deliver CAM treatments, whether conventional health professionals or CAM professionals, should have received training in that discipline independently accredited by the appropriate regulatory body.
>
> (House of Lords, 2000, para. 6.33)

While the growth in numbers of providers of CAM education and training seems to offer potential students additional choice, making an informed choice has become extremely difficult in a market where standards vary so widely.

2.4 Dilemmas in teaching CAM

Teaching CAM-related courses raises a range of interrelated issues about what should be taught, whether or not it is possible to teach CAM skills, and what sort of models of training are relevant to each modality. The fact that CAM is a diverse group of therapies (more than 200 according to Stone, 2002) means there will always be debate both within and among CAM therapies about whether modalities such as energy healing can be taught or whether they involve a high degree of inherent ability that cannot be learned.

ACTIVITY   CAN HEALING BE TAUGHT?

Allow about 10 minutes

Write a short paragraph in response to the question 'Can healing be taught?'

Comment

Many modalities make what could be called non-measurable claims about the qualities of their practitioners, such as 'intuition' or the ability to discern 'energy auras' around people. Moreover, some healers believe their ability to heal is a gift and that healing cannot be taught. This position is challenging to those who insist that what cannot be taught cannot be assessed and what cannot be assessed cannot be accredited. This is not to suggest that healing does not require certain distinct competencies, but rather that it involves skills that are hard to measure, or indeed, rationalise, such as transmitting the healing power of love.

CAM education raises important issues about how diverse notions of healing can be taught and examined within orthodox educational structures. Consequently, modalities such as healing require different forms of training than other forms of CAM that more closely resemble orthodox medicine. In the case of osteopathy, for instance, students can be examined on the principles of anatomy and physiology in the same way as students of orthodox medicine. Similarly, the practical application of skills in treating the body can be taught and evaluated through practical sessions and clinics, where teachers evaluate how successfully individual students can apply their modality. More esoteric CAM modalities demand different styles of teaching, learning and testing: for example, where healing forms part of indigenous traditions, a practitioner may acquire skills through familiarisation of sacred texts and induction by elders. Egan (1998) notes that in some approaches to therapeutic touch – a form of CAM that uses touch on or just above the body surface – knowing when and how to use it requires mentorship and practice. The modality is learned through an apprenticeship. In some methods of training this learning process depends on the individual and how long their learning experience takes until they are deemed ready to practise independently.

Degrees versus apprenticeships

CAM became more professionalised during the second half of the 20th century and training has increasingly been incorporated into HFE systems. Arguably, the key reason for this trend for incorporation is the drive towards increased integration of CAM in orthodox medical settings. There is also growing interest among orthodox health care staff in training in CAM and integrating it into their own practice. Whereas apprenticeship and mentorship are seen as valuable teaching methods in traditional healing systems, the training of health care practitioners in westernised cultures favours a large element of classroom-based academic training. Yet the HFE approach to training is not necessarily the best or only effective way of training competent CAM practitioners.

The cultural context of the therapy may have a significant impact on how new therapists are initiated or inducted into practice. Cassidy (1996) compared the training systems favoured by professional systems with how practitioners learn their craft in community-based systems. She found that in some other cultures healers enter apprenticeship by inheritance (birthright) or even by receiving a symbolic message or calling from god(s) or another world, indicating that the person has a 'natural' ability to be a healer. Rather than having a set time or curriculum to learn the skills to heal, training often only finishes when a mentor or master feels that the person is ready. Examinations, in the sense of the strict written tests familiar in the West, are often replaced by observation of the trainee healer's abilities and their acceptance as a healer by people in their own community. This shows that different models of teaching CAM have much to learn from other ways of training and are influenced by other cultures and other notions of what education and training should be about.

Apprenticeship models are unlikely to find favour in countries committed to broadening tertiary education. However, as Cassidy (1996) indicates, apprenticeship models recognise that a formal education may not be sufficient to guarantee that a graduate is competent. While much of a practitioner's technical knowledge may be gained at pre-registration level, the practical skills and wisdom required of a competent practitioner may take months or years of accumulated practical experience. Apprenticeships also seem to recognise that training should be seen as the beginning of a lifelong learning process situated within the community. Some of these ideals can be achieved in a non-apprenticeship model through integrating provisional periods of practice before qualifying as a fully registered practitioner; the use of CPD after registration and throughout the practitioner's working life; the encouragement of practitioner research; and revalidation processes.

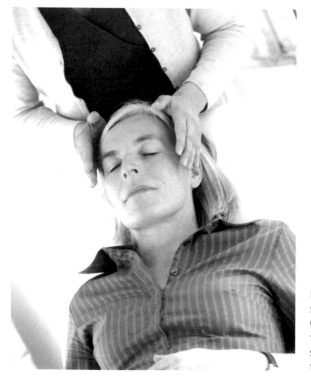

Reiki practitioners teach their students in a very direct way. Often the 'student' becomes the subject in order to learn some of the subtleties of the techniques

2.5   Debates in education and training

Level of biomedical knowledge required for safe CAM practice

The question of how much biomedical knowledge CAM practitioners need to practise safely is the subject of ongoing controversy. CAM practitioners who lack knowledge in medical science could miss serious underlying pathologies and treat patients inappropriately. CAM practitioners say this is a spurious argument, since they do not claim to make 'medical diagnoses' but offer treatment within an entirely different paradigm. Stone and Matthews (1996) suggest that, to comply with ethical requirements, a minimum level of biomedical knowledge is necessary:

> Although the amount of biomedical knowledge that practitioners require is the subject of fierce debate, a basic level of orthodox medical training is necessary for all practitioners so that, at the very least, they will be capable of recognizing contra-indications to their therapy and situations in which urgent, acute medical care is required. However unpalatable, we believe this is a necessary concomitant of complementary practitioners holding themselves out as providing therapies with specific health benefits. This may be assisted by co-operation with GMC [the General Medical Council] and Royal Colleges [of Medicine and Surgery, etc.] ... Because of the practical and philosophical problems in including a significant amount of biomedical knowledge in complementary therapists' training, and the problems which this raises in terms of practitioners' ability to spot serious underlying conditions which may require conventional treatment, therapists should be encouraged to work as closely alongside GPs as possible.
>
> (Stone and Matthews, 1996, p. 275)

A core curriculum for CAM?

The idea that all CAM modalities share a common basic curriculum might appear to be a good one at first sight. However, designing the content of a core curriculum for so many different types of therapy raises considerable difficulties and the idea has generally been unpopular within CAM. Objections have mostly been based on one of two arguments: either the scope of CAM disciplines is so diverse that to envisage a common body of knowledge that is useful for them all is too difficult; or people disagree on theoretical grounds with the concept of core curricula. In particular, the body representing universities – the CVCP (Committee of Vice Chancellors and Principals) – gave evidence to the House of Lords Committee, stating that they were against the inflexibility that a core curriculum across CAM might represent to individual universities and courses (House of Lords, 2000). While recognising the need for CAM regulatory bodies to define outcomes and standardise CAM education for each modality, the CVCP also supported the right of universities to define **how** they would get practitioners to agree to these outcomes.

ACTIVITY   DEVELOPING A CORE CURRICULUM: WHAT DO CAM PRACTITIONERS NEED TO KNOW?

Allow 20 minutes

The British Medical Association, the Foundation for Integrated Medicine (now the Prince of Wales's Foundation for Integrated Health) and the University of Westminster drew up the list of core curriculum subjects for CAM outlined in Box 2.2. Imagine you were contemplating visiting a herbalist and a crystal healer for chronic sinus problems. Which of the possible core curriculum subjects in Box 2.2 would you expect your practitioners to know about?

BOX 2.2   POSSIBLE CORE CURRICULUM SUBJECTS FOR CAM

- Basic biomedicine
- Fundamentals of conventional medical diagnosis and guidelines on patient referral
- CAM therapies and their potential uses, including the principles of diagnosis and practice
- Research methodology and the application of results
- Holistic models of health care
- Professional ethics
- The therapeutic relationship
- Clinical audit of outcomes
- Impact of social, cultural, economic, employment and environmental factors on health
- Counselling skills
- Principles of quality management and audit
- Organisational skills, including record keeping
- Technical skills, including information technology management

---

Comment

Some of the core curriculum subjects seem to be important to all practitioners: for example, professional ethics, an understanding of the therapeutic relationship and certainly good communication, if not counselling, skills. However, would you expect both the herbalist and the crystal healer to have a knowledge of basic biomedicine? Maybe basic biomedicine is helpful to a herbalist but it is harder to make a case for it to be part of a crystal healer's training. Other subjects on the list – such as research methodology, clinical audit of outcomes and the principles of quality management and audit – do not seem essential to either as individual practitioners, although both modalities need to draw on these competencies. In fact, the bodies who suggested the list of core curriculum subjects did not go as far as stipulating who should be expected to study all or any of them. Their intention was to begin the process of discussion around what kinds of shared knowledge base would be useful to the development of CAM.

Clearly, decisions about training are also entangled with issues of control over knowledge, professional integrity and the customs of the institutions involved in training. Traditionally, universities have a heritage of allowing much freedom in teaching and learning, thus the suggestion of a core curriculum sits awkwardly with these values. However, most professions (both inside and outside health) are increasingly looking to a competencies-based approach, which will tend to standardise how a subject is taught. A core curriculum across CAM, while providing opportunities for cross-fertilisation between modalities, may have insurmountable difficulties. The conclusion of the House of Lords report on this topic is that flexibility is needed for training settings and among providers:

> **We conclude that there should be flexibility for training institutions to decide how to educate practitioners.** To introduce one formal core curriculum across healthcare would be a Herculean task; there is no obvious body available to tackle such a task which, in any case, would no doubt meet with much opposition … **We do not advocate a blanket core curriculum.**
>
> (House of Lords, 2000, para. 6.61)

While a core curriculum is contentious, most interested parties see the development of core competencies as being useful. In effect this means, rather than creating an inflexible notion of what all CAM training should contain, the focus is more on developing common understandings that would enable CAM practitioners to work with other modalities or with a range of orthodox or integrated health care workers (Park, 2002).

Development of competencies and NOSs

The notion of 'competence' relates to the skills and abilities required of a practitioner in a given CAM. The point of defining competencies is that they represent agreement within the therapy about what constitutes the core elements of being able to practise that therapy in a safe and effective manner. Different training schools will continue to provide their own, even idiosyncratic, approach to training that will promote diversity within each modality. None the less, the establishment of core competencies is important to enable consolidation, promote cohesion and set out the minimum requirements for training and practice.

Ideally, collections of skills and abilities should be determined at a collective level by the profession as a whole. In order to determine training and practice standards, professional groups need to set aside differences and concentrate on their commonalities and shared philosophies. If competencies were developed in this way, there could be agreed differences to take account of the various therapeutic approaches within a given therapy, while ensuring basic levels of safety. The problem here is that, historically, only the most professionalised schools and associations become involved in defining competencies or discussing what should be included. Although politically active, these bodies may not be representative of the therapy as a whole. Any attempt to devise profession-wide competencies must try to ensure that as many different interest groups are consulted as possible.

As noted earlier, a fairly recent development within CAM is the creation of NOSs in several modalities. This is a developmental process and progress has been made towards having agreed standards within each CAM modality. However, the process has not been universally accepted in all of them. There are several problems involved in trying to bring together practitioners and professional organisations to agree set standards for each modality. As well as the temptation for consultation to involve only the largest or most vocal professional groups, there are the practical logistics of bringing together all the professional organisations and training providers in an inclusive way. It is easy for groups to be left out of the consultation process or to believe they are unheard during it. In addition, there are often divisions, not only over philosophical issues but also over how training should be carried out in a modality. A good example of this is the differences between schools of hypnotherapy: some favour a highly theoretical curriculum and long training; others emphasise the importance of hands-on learning, and yet others work solely on the basis of distance learning.

Such differences may usually be latent; however, the need to develop a framework can sometimes magnify disputes. For instance, in aromatherapy the standards that were developed were rejected by the Institute for Complementary Medicine, the British Register of Complementary Practitioners (Aromatherapy Division) and the International Federation of Aromatherapists because, they argued, the standards reflected the lowest level of competence. These groups thought the standards should aim higher and not be just about the bare minimum. Interestingly, these same NOSs were accepted by the Aromatherapy Organisations Council, the British Complementary Medicine Association and the Independent Care Organisations, which is now part of the Training Organisations for the Personal Social Services. This situation resulted in the QCA reviewing the NOSs in aromatherapy. The process of bringing different groups together can be creative and productive. It can allow different traditions of one modality to work together on commonalities as well as offer the opportunity to celebrate differences in tradition, style of working and philosophy.

Is there a need for continuing professional development?

If professional practice is to be safe and competent, there needs to be an understanding of how knowledge, skills and attitudes are evolving and how practice is changing. Professionals have an ethical duty to keep themselves up to date, so that they can offer what is currently regarded as best practice within their particular field and be prepared to adapt their own practice in the light of new evidence. This ability to respond to a changing environment is central to the concept of **lifelong learning**. This concept has been embraced by the NHS (Department of Health, 1999), where health professionals are required to maintain and develop their practice in order to move up through the relevant pay bands. Of course, the majority of CAM practitioners work in private practice, so may not be exposed to the same external pressures to keep their skills up to date. However, CPD involves a willingness to adopt and create innovative approaches to practice. A healer who originally trained and has practised independently for many years may have to acquire new skills in order to work in integrated health settings, such as working in a multidisciplinary team, keeping computerised records and auditing their practice. Professional practice now requires professionals to continue to develop their competence and expertise over the course of their career.

The formalised way in which professional learning becomes a lifelong process is through CPD. According to the House of Lords:

> Continuing Professional Development is vital if professionals are to keep up with new developments in their field; it is also a mechanism that can be used to encourage research understanding and inter-professional collaboration.
>
> (House of Lords, 2000, para. 6.34)

CPD involves more than technical competencies (see Box 2.3 overleaf). Whereas competence-based practice is externally driven and is about minimum standards for safe practice, CPD should be internally motivated, driven by the practitioner's desire for self-development. The UK government has introduced formal structures to ensure CPD throughout the NHS (Department of Health, 1999). The core principles it espouses could be applied to CPD in CAM.

The Osteopaths Act 1993 and the Chiropractors Act 1994 make specific provision for CPD as part of their statutory framework. CPD is slowly being introduced in homeopathy, herbalism and acupuncture, although, as with other areas of education and training, the type and the quality of the training vary significantly. In other therapies, a formalised requirement for CPD remains uncommon, although this situation is gradually changing.

> ### BOX 2.3   CORE PRINCIPLES OF CONTINUING PROFESSIONAL DEVELOPMENT
>
> CPD should be:
>
> - purposeful and patient-centred
> - participative, i.e. fully involving the individual and other relevant stakeholders
> - targeted at identified educational need
> - educationally effective
> - part of a wider organisational development plan in support of local and national service objectives
> - focused on the development needs of clinical teams, across traditional professional and service boundaries
> - designed to build on previous knowledge, skills and experience
> - designed to enhance the skills of interpreting and applying knowledge based on research and development.
>
> (Source: Department of Health, 1999, para. 3.1)

Who is going to organise CPD and who will pay for it? A coherent programme of CPD requires CAM professional bodies to devote considerable time and resources and the costs may be prohibitive for smaller professional bodies. Moreover, the notion of what CPD should involve varies among therapies. Whereas psychotherapists and counsellors may consider being in therapy themselves as a necessary aspect of their ongoing professional development, practitioners of oriental therapies such as shiatsu and acupuncture might believe that training in other oriental modalities such as t'ai chi or qi gong serves a similar function. Another factor is that while the 'Big Five' therapies may require many hours of formal CPD and skills updating, other modalities may consider five or six hours a year of more informal personal development as being acceptable. Indeed, the time spent overall on CPD may not be as important as the impact of the development. As Hugh MacPherson argues, deeper approaches to CPD:

> could recognise that personal development is often inextricably linked to one's development as a practitioner, that a shift in values can have a profound effect on the quality of one's practice, and that a growing awareness of ethics, say for example becoming aware of our prejudices, could significantly influence the way our practice grows.
>
> (MacPherson, 1995, p. 37)

For some modalities, extensive formal CPD may not be as useful as shorter periods of informal reflective work that emphasises personal growth. Another difficult issue is how CPD should be developed for people trained in multiple modalities. Certainly, extensive CPD for, say, a holistic practitioner who is trained and practises four different types of CAM may raise issues of finance and time constraints.

It is important that CPD feeds back into professional practice and is valued by practitioners. An obvious way to make CPD a higher priority for CAM practitioners is to link it with ongoing professional registration. For example, the General Medical Council (GMC) is in the process of introducing revalidation procedures which require orthodox practitioners to demonstrate CPD throughout their career in order to maintain their professional registration and ongoing licence to practise.

Cross-specialisation

The competence of CAM practitioners may be questioned when a practitioner who is trained in one therapy incorporates techniques from another therapy. It is very common for therapists to use a variety of therapeutic modalities when treating clients:

> Complementary practitioners, although usually having one major specialty, may use, comment on and recommend a very wide range of different treatment methods in routine clinical practice. The most widely used supplementary regimes are diet, exercise, vitamins, herbal remedies, massage and relaxation. These are core treatments drawn on by many practitioners.
>
> (Vincent and Furnham, 1997, p. 18)

The use of more than one therapeutic approach is ethically acceptable, **providing** practitioners are adequately trained in each modality they use. Of course, in a generally unregulated field, the issue of 'adequate' training is in itself problematic.

2.6   CAM familiarisation and training for orthodox practitioners

As the popularity of CAM has grown, there have been calls for more knowledge about it to be included in the training of orthodox health professionals. Currently, in both the UK and the USA, significant proportions of medical and nursing schools are offering students courses in CAM familiarisation or, in some cases, the basics of CAM modalities (Park, 2002).

ACTIVITY   CAM AWARENESS TRAINING FOR ORTHODOX PRACTITIONERS

Allow 15 minutes

Why might each of the orthodox practitioners listed below benefit from some form of CAM familiarisation?

1   A physiotherapist
2   A palliative care nurse
3   A general practitioner (GP)

Comment

A growing proportion of the population uses CAM so, at a general level, all orthodox practitioners need to know something about the CAM treatments that their patients may be using.

1   A physiotherapist would benefit from some understanding of osteopathy, chiropractic, acupuncture and therapeutic massage, all of which might be useful to their patients, particularly those with chronic back problems.

2   A palliative care nurse may benefit from understanding forms of pain relief developed in CAM therapies such as acupuncture. Spiritual healing may ease the pain of dying for some palliative care patients and aromatherapy massage can bring relief from generalised discomfort.

3   GPs are often consulted as a general source of information about health. Increasingly they may be asked for their views on nutritional supplements, the use of herbal remedies or the merits of acupuncture. GPs are the gatekeepers to NHS-provided CAM services, so they need to understand enough about CAM to know when a referral is appropriate.

CAM familiarisation as a precursor of integration

To achieve greater integration between CAM and orthodox medicine, it could be argued that CAM practitioners should become familiar with biomedical types of diagnostic procedures and treatments, and that orthodox practitioners should improve their awareness of the available CAM treatments. The GMC (2003) supports greater familiarisation of CAM approaches for orthodox health professionals at both undergraduate and postgraduate levels. There is a crucial distinction between courses aimed at familiarising orthodox practitioners with CAM, so they can advise patients about which CAM therapies they might find helpful, and courses intended to equip practitioners to offer CAM treatments themselves. In the latter case, the government supports the training of orthodox health care practitioners to standards agreed with an appropriate (single) CAM regulatory body.

The need for CAM familiarisation has also been recognised by the GMC:

> [Graduates] must be aware that many patients are interested in and choose to use a range of alternative and complementary therapies. Graduates must be aware of the existence and range of such therapies, why some patients use them, and how these might affect other types of treatment that patients are receiving.
>
> (GMC, 2003, p. 6, para. 18)

What form should CAM familiarisation take?

The report of the House of Lords Select Committee (2000) found that the current provision of CAM familiarisation in medical schools was haphazard and varied considerably among different schools. CAM familiarisation occurred in two main ways: a little information was offered in the general curriculum and there was an option of more specialised study, for students who are interested, in the form of an optional 'special study module'. The House of Lords recommended that every medical school includes a level of CAM familiarisation for all their medical undergraduates that makes them aware of their patients' possible choices. It also recommended a similar approach for the nursing curriculum. While this dealt with familiarisation, the House of Lords noted that orthodox health care practitioners who want to go beyond familiarisation and incorporate CAM into their own practice should seek specific training at postgraduate level (para. 6.86).

2.7   Conclusion

Issues concerning the education and training of CAM practitioners are a challenge to people who want to see all CAM therapies develop their professional status and raise their standards. Clearly, a key problem in improving standards is the range and diversity of CAM modalities and their educational heritage. For some practitioners, CAM education has been based on charismatic teaching, with perhaps little theoretical or formal background. For others, training has developed into a broader educational process, with strict entrance procedures, formal classes, examinations and the award of a degree upon successful completion. The introduction of National Occupational Standards in complementary therapy, the move within many CAM regulatory bodies to at least stipulate and monitor basic educational standards, and the increasing focus on continuing professional development suggest a growing awareness within the sector that good education and training are essential for competent and safe practice.

KEY POINTS

- Education and training within CAM have become more professionalised in recent years and, in the case of some of the 'Big Five' therapies, are comparable to the education and training of orthodox health care practitioners.

- Within less well established therapies, there is an unacceptable diversity in the levels and standards of training offered.

- There is a movement within CAM away from charismatic training and private sector provision towards externally validated training within more formal higher education systems.

- Most CAM courses include a level of biomedical knowledge and many orthodox medical practitioners now have some level of CAM familiarisation in their training.

- Continuing professional development is recognised as being essential to the ongoing development of CAM practitioners, but regulatory bodies vary in the extent to which they require it.

References

Bakx, K. (1991) 'The eclipse of folk medicine in Western society', *Sociology of Health and Illness*, Vol. 13, No. 1, pp. 20–38.

British Medical Association (1993) *Complementary Medicine: New Approaches to Good Practice*, London, BMA.

Cant, S. (1996) 'From charismatic teaching to professional training: the legitimation of knowledge and the creation of trust in homoeopathy and chiropractic', in Cant, S. and Sharma, U. (eds) *Complementary and Alternative Medicines: Knowledge in Practice*, London, Free Association Books.

Cassidy, C. M. (1996) 'Cultural context of complementary and alternative medicine systems', in Micozzi, M. (ed.) *Fundamentals of Complementary and Alternative Medicine*, Edinburgh, Churchill Livingstone.

Chamberlain, M. (1982) *Old Wives' Tales*, London, Virago.

Department of Health (1999) *Continuing Professional Development: Quality in the New NHS*, London, The Stationery Office.

Dobraszczyc, U. (1989) *Sickness, Health, and Medicine*, London, Longman.

Egan, E. C. (1998) 'Therapeutic touch', in Snyder, M. and Lindquist, R. (eds) *Complementary and Alternative Therapies in Nursing* (3rd edition), Berlin, Springer Publishing Company Inc.

General Medical Council (2003) *Tomorrow's Doctors*, London, GMC.

House of Lords (2000) Sixth Report of the House of Lords Science and Technology Committee, *Complementary and Alternative Medicine*, London, The Stationery Office.

MacPherson, H. (1995) 'Great talents ripen late: continuing education in the acupuncture profession', *European Journal of Oriental Medicine*, Vol. 1, No. 6, pp. 35–9.

Nicholls, P. (2005) 'Homoeopathy, hospitals and high society', in Lee-Treweek, G., Heller, T., Spurr, S., MacQueen, H. and Katz, J. (eds) *Perspectives on Complementary and Alternative Medicine: A Reader*, pp. 203–10, Abingdon, Routledge/The Open University (K221 Set Book).

Park, C. (2002) 'Diversity, the individual, and proof of efficacy: complementary and alternative medicine in medical education', *American Journal of Public Health*, Vol. 92, No. 10, pp. 1568–72.

Porter, R. (1999) *The Greatest Benefit to Mankind: A Medical History of Humanity from Antiquity to the Present*, London, Fontana.

Rankin-Box, D. (2001) *Nurses' Handbook of Complementary Therapies* (2nd edition), London, Baillière-Tindall.

Skills for Health (2003) Website: www.skillsforhealth.org [accessed 3 August 2004].

Stone, J. (2002) *An Ethical Framework for Complementary and Alternative Therapists*, London, Routledge.

Stone, J. and Matthews, J. (1996) *Complementary Medicine and the Law*, Oxford, Oxford University Press.

Vincent, C. and Furnham, A. (1997) *Complementary Medicine: A Research Perspective*, Chichester, John Wiley & Sons.

Chapter 3 Regulation and control

Julie Stone and Geraldine Lee-Treweek

Contents

AIMS

■ To review the issues around the regulation and control of CAM therapies.

■ To outline some of the problems and possibilities of the practical implementation of regulating CAM.

3.1 Introduction

Health care in the UK is a highly regulated activity. Whereas the orthodox medical profession has been statutorily regulated for over 150 years, most therapies in complementary and alternative medicine (CAM) remain unregulated or are regulated voluntarily. More recently, the government has imposed stricter regulation across the range of health care professions to meet the primary goal of regulation, which is to protect the public (Department of Health, 2001a).

Since the second half of the 1990s, the government has introduced numerous measures to meet concerns over public safety after several highly publicised incidences of serious malpractice and de facto regulatory failures within the field of orthodox medical and social work practice. This includes examples where individual practitioners, such as Beverley Allitt and Harold Shipman, committed serious illegal acts using their professional position to the detriment of members of the general public. There are also examples of institutional failure, such as within the paediatric cardiac surgery unit at the

Bristol Royal Infirmary. In response to the official inquiry (Kennedy, 2001), the government created several new bodies, including the Council for the Regulation of Healthcare Professionals, to improve patient safety through better regulation. While most CAM is practised outside the National Health Service (NHS), there have also been regulatory advances in the CAM sector. There have been calls for improved regulation from consumers, doctors and therapists themselves (Mills, 2001). Most therapies are moving towards a single professional body for each profession (White, 2004), and many CAM-related therapeutic organisations have been improving their voluntary regulatory structures. The motivations for seeking regulation are complex. In addition to improving patient protection, regulation can also enhance professional status and respectability. After the creation of the General Osteopathic Council in 1993 and the General Chiropractic Council in 1994, other CAM therapies have undergone significant professionalisation with the intention of pursuing statutory regulation. Chapter 4 deals with the issue of professionalisation in greater depth.

The form of regulation most commonly sought up until now is **statutory self-regulation** (SSR). The model for this is the Medical Act 1858, which established the orthodox medical practitioners' own body, the General Medical Council (GMC). This is an example of professional self-regulation in which a profession sets its own standards and monitors its own performance, while being ultimately answerable to a branch of government known as the Privy Council. This form of regulation is financed entirely by the profession itself through annual fees paid by registered therapists. Although most CAM therapies aspire to SSR, it may not be the most appropriate form of regulation for all of them. For small therapies that do not pose a risk of harm to users, the cost of SSR may be disproportionate to the inherent risk of the therapy.

The government tends to consider granting autonomous SSR only to therapies of proven efficacy, which already have effective voluntary regulatory mechanisms in place. In general terms, the government supports a hands-off regulatory approach and does not encourage disproportionate regulation. The government only intervenes to impose statutory regulation if it believes the public cannot be adequately protected through less burdensome means.

This chapter will show that regulation, especially in the form of statutory self-regulation, is not a panacea. Regulatory mechanisms are only effective if they are relevant, up to date, and properly enforced. The future integration of CAM with orthodox medicine will not necessarily depend on statutory regulation, even though this may be cited as another reason to pursue regulation. Furthermore, the statutory regulation of a CAM therapy does not guarantee that the therapy will be widely adopted within the NHS. While some CAM practitioners view statutory regulation as a means of enhancing their profession, others see it as a slippery slope to unwanted control and interference by the government. Unless sensitively managed, the transition from voluntary self-regulation (VSR) to SSR may alienate the fundamental membership of a CAM therapy. If this happens, practitioners may resist formal regulation, even when it is imposed on them.

3.2   What is 'regulation'?

Moran and Wood (1993, p. 17) define regulation as **'the activity by which the rules governing the exchange of goods and services are made and implemented'**. The primary purpose of regulation is to protect the public. Health care regulation seeks to ensure that practitioners have had appropriate training and are competent to practise and work within certain ethical standards. The main premise of professional self-regulation is that professional practice is based on highly technical skills and that, as a result, the profession is best suited to set its standards and monitor professional performance against those standards.

Despite the explicit purpose of public protection, there is the key question of whether professional groups seeking regulation are motivated predominantly by public interest or by self-interest. Regulation can be described as a form of 'social closure'. This involves drawing a boundary around specialised knowledge and creating a monopoly through registration which lets some people in but excludes outsiders. Allsop and Saks (2002, p. 4) point out that this regulatory bargain between a profession and the state 'is not struck automatically or without a struggle. Rather, it is won through political engagement.'

Achieving professional status implies certain privileges. The market control that regulation ensures 'is associated with enhanced income, status and power, as well as self-regulation – in which the professional body has the responsibility to police itself, not least through the adoption of ethical and disciplinary codes' (Allsop and Saks, 2002, p. 5).

It is hard to assess how far self-interest drives the pursuit of regulation. For emerging professions, part of the motivation for seeking statutory regulation appears to be the increased prestige which practitioners believe this status will confer. Although usually presented as polarised positions, professional self-interest is not necessarily incompatible with public interest, and a stronger professional base can benefit both patients and practitioners (for example, by imposing stricter training standards on practitioners). The tension between these two concepts may be more pronounced in therapies where the regulator is charged with both the protection of the public and the promotion of the profession (as is the case with the Osteopaths Act 1993 and the Chiropractors Act 1994). Box 3.1 sets out the 'principles of good regulation' which were identified by the Better Regulation Task Force (2000), a Cabinet Office think-tank.

BOX 3.1   KEY PRINCIPLES OF REGULATION

1 **Transparency:** a clear definition of powers and rules, clear guidance to those affected by regulation, consultation over regulatory proposals, and openness about any regulatory failure that may occur.

2 **Accountability:** a clear mechanism of accountability to government, Parliament, the public and those who are being regulated, including an appeals system for the latter.

3 **Targeting:** a clear definition of goals, the targeting of regulatory efforts, the avoidance of universal approaches, flexibility of enforcement, and the modification or elimination of regulations shown to be ineffective or outdated.

4 **Consistency:** compatibility of written rules with the activities of other regulators and existing regulations, consistency with European Union and international trade policy, and consistency in enforcement by the relevant authorities at local level.

5 **Proportionality:** penalties for breaking rules should be appropriate, with measurement of the impact of regulation to establish the balance between risk and cost and the consideration of alternatives to state regulation.

The five principles outlined in Box 3.1 underpin the processes of the statutory health care regulators. They aim to protect the public while at the same time ensuring that the form of regulation is not unnecessarily burdensome on those being regulated. Statutory functions (including registration, standard setting and fitness to practise procedures) are checked against these five principles. Self-regulation does not operate in a vacuum, but within a broader framework of consumer and health and safety at work legislation.

ACTIVITY   OTHER CHECKS AND CONTROLS

Allow 10 minutes

How would you respond to the following questions?

- What other checks and controls are there on health care workers in the NHS?
- What redress do CAM users have without statutory regulations?

Comment

In the case of health care in the NHS, members of the public are protected from malpractice by the complaints system, employment and disciplinary procedures, clinical audit and clinical governance (Allsop and Mulcahy, 1996). All professional activity operates against the backdrop of general legal principles, thus users of CAM can sue their therapists if their work falls below acceptable standards. The law applies regardless of whether practitioners are statutorily regulated, voluntarily regulated or working in an entirely unaffiliated manner. However, it may not operate as well as more direct regulation.

Legal controls operate retrospectively and, particularly in the case of criminal and civil law, are probably only invoked when a user has already been harmed. As a preventive strategy, the law does little to protect people from harm or to raise standards within a profession generally (Stone and Matthews, 1995). From the consumer perspective, these coexisting complaints mechanisms may appear to be disjointed and confusing. This is compounded by poor referral mechanisms among different agencies. The role of the regulator may also be poorly understood, as a result of which regulators could receive complaints which fall outside their remit. One reason why regulators have acquired the image of being unhelpful and protectionist is because previously they have not supported complainants by redirecting mistargeted complaints to more appropriate channels. This may result in legitimate complaints not being heard.

3.3   The regulation of health care

Historically, health care professionals in the UK have been given a considerable amount of freedom in terms of how they establish themselves in a clinical setting and their ability to work autonomously (Price, 2002).

> The Common Law right to practise medicine means that in the United Kingdom anyone can treat a sick person even if they have no training in any type of healthcare whatsoever, provided that the individual treated has given informed consent ... Persons exercising this right must not identify themselves by any of the titles protected by statute and they cannot prescribe medicines that are regulated prescription-only drugs ... The Common Law right to practise springs from the fundamental principle that everyone can choose the form of healthcare that they require.
>
> (House of Lords, 2000, para. 5.9)

This laissez-faire approach to regulation has historical roots. Within conventional medicine, internalised controls such as the integrity and character of the physician were regarded as the principal ingredients of competent and appropriate patient care (Price, 2002). However, various trends suggest that this optimism is insufficient to protect patients from physical or psychological harm, including:

- increasing levels of complaints and litigation against health care practitioners
- evidence of professional abuse across all health and social care professions
- government insistence on greater professional accountability, transparency and openness
- changing attitudes towards professional authority
- increasing awareness of people's rights when they use health services
- improved access to information, potentially diminishing the knowledge differential between 'experts' and 'patients'.

The scope of health care regulation

In the UK, SSR is the preferred mechanism for governing health professionals. The key feature of SSR is that it protects certain professional titles. For example, it is a criminal offence for unsuitably qualified people to call themselves a doctor, nurse, midwife, chiropractor or an osteopath. Statutes which protect titles do not necessarily prohibit other people from carrying out the tasks associated with that title – they only prevent them from using the title. Certain professions in the UK, such as dentistry and health professions in other jurisdictions, protect professional function as well as title. Thus, the law prohibits people not only from calling themselves a dentist if they are not but also from practising dentistry. This **functional closure** has the effect of freezing the regulated activity, which makes it an inflexible form of regulation. The protection of function is necessarily restrictive and inflexible. It is only appropriate where functions can be defined unambiguously; are unlikely to change; and where all interested parties accept that the functions are unlikely to become appropriate for others to undertake (JM Consulting, 1998).

Price (2002) argues that protection of function is not conducive to fluidity in terms of allocating tasks and roles. He goes on to argue that protection of function runs counter to the government's recent commitment to expand the role that allied health professionals play in health and social care, allowing them to use their skills flexibly and creatively for the benefit of the patient (Department of Health, 2001b). What tends to happen is that a sub-profession arises, for example dental hygienists.

Although most people associate professional regulation predominantly with professional conduct and fitness to practise proceedings, the scope of health care regulation is considerably broader. As well as fitness to practise, regulators have a pivotal role in setting pre-registration standards and continuing professional development (CPD) requirements. According to Stone and Matthews (1995) health care regulation includes:

- registration of competent practitioners and protection of title (prosecuting people who use a professional title when they are not registered)
- effective fitness-to-practise procedures capable of administering constructive sanctions, ultimately including deregistration ('erasure') of practitioners who are a danger to patients
- mechanisms for providing compensation for harm (for example, the requirement for registered practitioners to carry indemnity insurance)
- access to dispute-resolving mechanisms other than the courts
- enforcement of high, uniform standards of pre-registration (and sometimes post-registration) education and training, and CPD
- protection of the public against exaggerated and false claims
- accountability, with clear procedures ensuring public confidence that consumer views and grievances will receive an effective response.

These are essentially the core functions of any system of self-regulation, whether it is voluntary or statutory. Taken in conjunction, these features are considered necessary to ensure that patients who consult professionals are adequately protected from harm. Although professional self-regulation may, at the same time, enhance the status and privileges of the protected group (for example, by bestowing certain professional privileges and creating a monopoly over who may practise that therapy), these should be considered secondary benefits.

Developments in health care regulation

Several highly publicised inquiries have revealed some of the shortcomings of self-regulation in the field of orthodox health care: in particular, the Kennedy Report on the Bristol Royal Infirmary Inquiry (Kennedy, 2001) and the Alder Hey Inquiry on tissue retention (Redfern, 2001). This has led to the development of various centralised initiatives designed to raise and maintain clinical standards in the NHS, including, for the first time, a statutory duty of care towards patients, and further development of the commitment to quality through the concept of clinical governance (Department of Health, 1997).

In addition, many arms-length regulatory bodies have been established to further protect patients through raised standards. These include the Healthcare Commission (formerly the Commission for Healthcare Audit and Inspection or CHAI), the National Patient Safety Agency (NPSA), the National Institute for Clinical Excellence (NICE), the National Clinical Assessment Authority (NCAA), and a new overarching statutory body – the Council for the Regulation of Healthcare Professionals (CRHP), since renamed the Council for Healthcare Regulatory Excellence (CHRE). The latter came into being in April 2003 and has far-reaching statutory powers to improve the functioning of health care regulatory bodies and to promote consistency among the bodies which regulate health care professionals. Against a backdrop of clinical governance and evidence-based medicine, health care professionals working within the NHS are now subject to several overlapping schemes of accountability.

Further changes were also introduced to the way in which individual health professions are regulated (Department of Health, 2001a, c). Extensive regulatory reforms were introduced in the practice of orthodox medicine (including the creation of revalidation procedures and a slimmed-down GMC, which has also increased its lay membership); in nursing, midwifery and health visiting (replacement of the United Kingdom Central Council or UKCC with the Nursing and Midwifery Council or NMC); and in the professions allied to medicine (replacement of the Council for Professions Supplementary to Medicine with a new Health Professions Council or HPC). Existing, arcane structures have been swept away and replaced with mechanisms which aim to promote greater accountability and transparency

(Allsop and Saks, 2002). Legislative changes have also been made to improve the regulatory schemes governing dentistry, pharmacy and ophthalmic practice.

Since 2000, all regulatory bodies have been encouraged to increase the proportion of lay representatives on their statutory committees. In a disciplinary context, this means having not only substantial lay representation on professional conduct committees but also a lay presence on the professional investigating committee which decides whether a case will be forwarded to the professional conduct committee.

ACTIVITY	THE IMPORTANCE OF A LAY PRESENCE IN PROFESSIONAL REGULATION

Allow 15 minutes

Briefly argue the case for and against having a lay presence in professional regulatory bodies.

Comment

In the past it was argued that, because of the highly technical nature of much of the work of health care professionals, regulatory bodies should consist of members of the given profession, especially when addressing matters of misconduct. It was thought that practitioners whose conduct was called into question should be judged by their peers because only similarly trained professionals could assess whether the alleged actions constituted professional misconduct. However, not all matters of misconduct involve technical decisions. In fact, the majority of professional misconduct cases turn on issues of ethical propriety, so professional peers may be less well suited to judge professional misconduct than independent lay members. The lay public is now much better informed and lay representatives do not have a vested interest in protecting their peers or their profession; indeed, their role is to protect the public interest. Of course, there are questions about how lay representatives are chosen and just how representative of the general public they are. However, some lay representation is better than no lay representation and should go a little way to increase transparency and accountability, which are two of the five key principles of regulation identified by the Better Regulation Task Force (see Box 3.1).

3.4 The challenge of regulating CAM

If CAM was once thought of as a marginal health care activity, clearly the government now recognises that it has a role to play in the delivery of modern health care. However, the credibility of CAM increasingly depends on its ability to embrace the principles of best practice in health care regulation. How has CAM responded to this regulatory challenge?

The scope of CAM therapists to practise CAM therapies and CAM patients to receive them largely depends on how these therapies fit in with the government's overall health strategies. Changing political climates therefore have a direct impact on the regulation of CAM. A free-market economy stressing decentralisation and deregulation is unlikely to impose excessive restraints on which therapies are offered and how they are regulated. In terms of health, governments which are trying to reduce public spending tend to highlight the 'virtues' of independence and self-reliance and so may look favourably on complementary therapies which promote self-healing and people taking personal responsibility for their health and wellbeing.

In its response to the House of Lords Report, the government highlights the fact that CAM has flourished in a hands-off regulatory environment:

> There has been increased public interest in and use of CAM in recent years. CAM is a thriving feature of the private healthcare sector, and may owe some of its commercial success to the fact that it currently enjoys relatively light regulation. The Government's overall policy towards better regulation is that it should be both proportionate and effective. In other words, the regulation should give customers adequate protection, without stifling the commercial services they want.
>
> (Department of Health, 2001d, p. 3)

In much of Europe, CAM practice is restricted to registered medical practitioners. Fears of European harmonisation have fuelled moves by UK practitioners towards professionalisation and the pursuit of statutory recognition. Despite freedom-of-movement directives and mutual recognition of qualifications, the law governing each member state will prevail domestically, including several highly restrictive regimes in which the practice of medicine (broadly defined so as to include CAM activities) is restricted to registered medical practitioners. Thus, despite the high use of CAM in many European Union countries, formally it has to be delivered by doctors since all lay practice is unlawful (and thus technically capable of prosecution). None the less, the recognition of the individual right to choice in health care is a view that has also been gaining ground throughout Europe.

In the Netherlands, a Commission for Alternative Systems of Medicine (1981) found that the consensus of public opinion was no longer behind the medical monopoly that existed at that time. In their opinion, the law was frequently being broken as sick and disabled people sought the help of people who were not legally authorised to provide it.

In the USA, the battle between CAM practitioners and doctors has been even more overt than in the UK, and the medical establishment actively prohibited association between doctors and 'irregulars'. Currently, most therapies are subject to strict licensing, with state licensing boards setting out training requirements and the scope of practice (Cohen, 1998).

Even governments which previously adopted a laissez-faire approach towards CAM may feel compelled to take a more interventionist stance if new trends emerge. These might include evidence showing that patients are being harmed by CAM; that CAM is expanding beyond its present boundaries and offering a viable alternative to seriously ill patients; or that CAM is growing to such an extent that it becomes a significant economic threat to drug-based conventional medicine.

The lack of overarching, effective regulation in CAM means that in unregulated therapies users could be consulting therapists who:

- may belong to any one of several competing professional registers or to none at all
- may belong to a professional body which has a wholly ineffective complaints set-up, or no complaints mechanism at all
- may or may not have had adequate training or be in possession of suitable professional skills
- may or may not carry any insurance in the event of something going seriously wrong.

People appear to use CAM therapies regardless of whether they are well regulated or not, which places them at potential risk of harm. In the UK, consumer freedom has historically been valued over consumer protection. This means that service users have the widest choice over who they may consult, but they may have a reduced degree of protection if something goes wrong.

ACTIVITY   CHECKING YOUR THERAPIST'S CREDENTIALS

Allow 15 minutes

If you have ever consulted a CAM therapist, did you check their credentials before you committed yourself to their care?

1   Did you find out about their actual qualifications?
2   Did you know whether their modality was subject to regulation?

If you have never consulted a CAM therapist, imagine you are going to. How would you find the answers to questions (1) and (2)?

Comment

It can be quite daunting to find out about qualifications and regulation. Letters after the therapist's name are one indication but they are often difficult to decipher. If you have consulted a CAM therapist you may well not have actively checked their credentials. Like many people, you probably consulted on a friend's recommendation or perhaps the therapist operated in a group whose reputation locally was sound. People do not usually enter a therapeutic relationship expecting anything to go wrong. Most users do not check a practitioner's credentials when they start therapy and they may simply assume that any therapist they consult has had suitable training and is competent to practise. This degree of trust is not necessarily misplaced, as most practitioners are highly committed to their clients and practitioners are individually accountable.

Statutory self-regulation and voluntary self-regulation in CAM

As noted in the introduction, CAM modalities range from having no regulation to voluntary self-regulation (VSR) or full statutory self-regulation (SSR).

The main difference between a voluntary scheme and a statutory scheme is the extent to which the professional body can enforce the standards it sets. This partly turns on the question of **protection of title**, which was discussed in Section 3.3. In a statutory scheme, the ability to use a professional title is limited to people who are properly included on a professional register maintained by the professional body, having had an appropriate level of training. Osteopathy and chiropractic are examples of therapies with protection of title. This means that, since the Osteopaths Act 1993 and the Chiropractors Act 1994 came into force, it is a criminal offence to use the title 'osteopath' or chiropractor' without being on the relevant statutory register.

Therapies which try to move from VSR to SSR face several potential problems. Some therapists may frustrate the purposes of the Act by refusing to join the statutory register or, having not been admitted on to a register, continuing to practise. The House of Lords report notes that some former osteopathic practitioners who were refused registration under the Osteopaths Act have continued to practise as 'osteomyologists', 'cranio-sacral practitioners', or other titles which are not protected under the Act. In this way, they frustrated the purposes of the Act, since it protects only titles, not functions (Price, 2002).

Midwifery and dentistry are professions in which both the professional title **and** the professional function are protected. For example, it is unlawful for anyone other than a registered midwife to attend to a woman in childbirth (other than in an emergency). Protection of function is not practical for CAM because of the broad range of practitioners who use different therapies (for example, physiotherapists who use acupuncture or nurses who use aromatherapy) and the tendency of therapists to cross-specialise, combining several therapeutic modalities.

The main concern about VSR is the enforceability of professional standards. Can voluntary regulation adequately protect members of the public from harm? In a voluntarily regulated therapy, while there are great advantages to belonging to a professional body, therapists cannot be forced to register. This is strongly the case in fitness-to-practise functions but is just as relevant to training and CPD requirements. There are difficulties in making self-employed, self-funding practitioners have extensive and ongoing training but practitioners who fail to keep up to date are a serious concern to public safety.

Criteria for regulating CAM

Clearly, it is unhelpful to talk about CAM as though it were a single, discrete entity. The regulatory requirements of CAM vary enormously from therapy to therapy. It is not easy to determine what level of regulation is appropriate. The criteria could include: whether the therapy puts the patient at risk of direct harm; whether the therapy is inherently low risk but could be risky if practised by non-medically trained staff; how long-standing the therapy is; and practitioners' level of training. Another possible criterion is how closely the therapy resembles another modality already provided within the NHS (for example, nutritional therapy is unregulated, whereas dietetics is regulated under the Health Professions Council). As in other areas of regulation, a distinction has been drawn between **complementary therapies** (which may be provided alongside conventional medicine) and **alternative therapies** (which purport to offer diagnostic information as well as therapy), the latter being seen as more in need of regulation.

House of Lords' criteria for regulating CAM

The House of Lords report suggests that a three-tier grouping of therapies should be applied to regulating CAM.

The first group, usually considered to be the 'Big Five', embraces the principal disciplines, two of which – osteopathy and chiropractic – are already regulated in their professional practice and training by Acts of Parliament. The others are acupuncture, herbal medicine and homeopathy. Each therapy claims to have an individual diagnostic approach.

The second group of therapies comprises those used most often to complement conventional medicine and does not purport to embrace diagnostic skills. This group includes aromatherapy; the Alexander Technique; body work therapies, including massage; counselling; stress therapy; hypnotherapy; reflexology and probably shiatsu; meditation; and healing.

The third group covers those disciplines purporting to offer diagnostic information as well as treatment. In general, they favour a philosophical approach, which is indifferent to the scientific principles of orthodox medicine, and proposes various disparate frameworks of disease causation and its management. These therapies can be split into two sub-groups. Group 3a includes long-established and traditional systems of health care such as ayurvedic medicine and traditional Chinese medicine. Group 3b covers other alternative disciplines which lack any significant evidence base, such as crystal therapy, iridology, radionics, dowsing and kinesiology (House of Lords, 2000).

The House of Lords determined that the therapies in Groups 2 and 3 did not require statutory regulation:

> A good voluntary regulatory structure is needed before a profession can seek statutory regulatory status. None of the therapies in Groups 2 and 3 has yet united under one professional body, and so statutory regulation is not a viable option for them at the present time. Indeed, for the disciplines we have listed in Group 3, such a prospect seems to us remote. For therapies in Group 2 the inherent risks of the therapies are minimal, and most are used as a complement to conventional medicine and not as an alternative, but to ensure that the public are protected from rogue practitioners, and have clear reliable information on these therapies, a good voluntary regulatory structure would be of benefit. Therefore, we recommend that practitioners of each of the therapies in Group 2 should organise themselves under a single professional body for each therapy. These bodies should be well-promoted so that the public who access these therapies are aware of them. Each should comply with core professional principles, and relevant information about each body should be made known to medical practitioners and other healthcare professionals. Patients could then have a single, reliable point of reference for standards, and would be protected against the risk of poorly-trained practitioners and have redress for poor service.
>
> (House of Lords, 2000, para. 5.23)

Despite the House of Lords' view that effective VSR should be sufficient to protect the public in the case of most CAM therapies, calls for tighter regulation persist. The response from CAM practitioners is not unified. However, as Stone (1996) notes, there is a substantial body of CAM therapists who, following on from osteopaths in 1993 and chiropractors in 1994, aspire to achieve SSR in a similar form to the Medical Act 1983. Stone suggests they might hope to gain:

- the medical profession's respect, together with a greater willingness to refer patients to complementary therapists
- improved prospects of integration within the NHS
- the ability to achieve higher standards and greater accountability through a system of statutory registration
- enhanced public status.

Stone (1996) goes on to question whether these assumptions are realistic. She points out that medical respect and employment within the NHS are based on cost-effectiveness and clinical efficacy as well as consumer demand. Similarly, public respect is gained more through therapeutic competence, ethical codes of conduct and rigorous complaints procedures, none of which are guaranteed by SSR. Whether it is desirable or not, is greater regulation a viable goal for CAM?

The response of CAM to the challenge of regulation

In the past, CAM was characterised by unhelpful professional fragmentation. Historically, CAM professional groups failed to negotiate effectively with each other, and far less to negotiate with statutory authorities, the medical profession or other interested parties. The sector included vocal and forceful personalities, and regulatory progress was hindered by infighting among competing professional groups. In addition, the growth of numerous self-styled umbrella bodies, straddling regulatory and quasi trade union functions, complicated matters further. Commenting on this unacceptable state of affairs, in its response to the House of Lords report, the government repeated the British Medical Association's call in 1993 for therapies to unite to protect patients:

> The Government believes professional self-regulation works best when it operates as an open and transparent partnership between the profession, patients and the wider public. These stakeholders clearly deserve better than the current fragmented regulation of certain CAM therapies. The Government therefore strongly encourages the regulating bodies within each therapy to unite to form a single body to regulate each profession. We believe this approach will be in the best interests of patients and the wider public, as well as potentially enhancing the status of individual professions.
>
> (Department of Health, 2001d, p. 7)

The multiplicity of professional registers continues to be of particular concern to public safety. It can be hard to assess the quality of a practitioner's training simply by noting the letters after their name. Furthermore, expulsion from one register provides inadequate patient protection if a practitioner who has been 'erased' or suspended by one professional body can simply apply to join a different register within the same therapy.

This situation is improving considerably, as CAM modalities move towards greater professionalisation. Most therapies have come together under a single regulatory body for each modality. The Prince of Wales's Foundation for Integrated Health, funded by a £1 million King's Fund award, set up several regulatory working groups, each steered by an independent chairperson, to carry this agenda forward. Increasingly significant proportions of therapists are registered with credible regulatory bodies, many of whom co-operate at national level to ensure consistent standards for training and practice. In addition, consumer awareness is growing, so that people are more likely to consult practitioners who belong to a recognised professional body.

None the less, groups of CAM practitioners remain who are implacably opposed to any form of external regulation.

For some CAM practitioners, the question is not how CAM should be regulated but **whether CAM is even amenable to formal regulation**. The government has stated that it will only consider regulation of therapies that can demonstrate the efficacy of their treatments. In effect this means only therapies that can demonstrate effectiveness in scientific terms will stand a chance of gaining statutory recognition. In order to demonstrate this sort of efficacy, a therapy must be able to produce research of a standard that is acceptable to the scientific community. Wherever possible, this is in the form of randomised controlled trials (RCTs). This overlooks the methodological difficulties of applying RCTs to holistic therapies, and the fact that most major research-funding bodies are reluctant to fund significant studies of complementary therapies.

The requirement for a therapy to prove itself in scientific terms almost certainly rules out the validation of many therapies, particularly spiritual, energy or vibrational therapies, which may not be amenable to being studied in ways that most scientists would find acceptable. It is not coincidental that the CAM modalities which have sought, or are seeking, statutory regulation have become more 'scientific' in their outlook. Therapists who reject the idea of pandering to the requirements of the orthodox biomedical view continue to be concerned about the extent to which the pursuit of statutory regulation could end up changing the nature of their therapeutic practice. As Stone (1996, p. 1493) points out, 'many therapists are not prepared to sacrifice their therapeutic integrity to validate themselves within a scientific paradigm. To do so would, in the view of many therapists, be to create a medicalised version of the therapy, denying its philosophical underpinnings.'

Other therapists view regulation as an unwarranted restriction of their autonomy. Many private CAM practitioners, who currently enjoy a high level of professional freedom, have little interest in what general practitioners think about them, and have no interest in working within the NHS. They would certainly resent the role of GPs as gatekeepers to their professional services. For this reason many of them tend to steer clear of regulatory debates. So the picture is very complex, with some modalities actively seeking regulation, while others are directly opposed.

3.5   The consequences of statutory and voluntary regulation of CAM

For CAM practitioners

Most CAM practitioners accept that, despite the evidence of their growing popularity, their continuing market share depends on them being perceived as professional. This means being registered by an appropriate regulatory body, being bound by its code of ethics and fitness-to-practise mechanisms, and maintaining appropriate insurance, so that patients are assured of a high level of safety and service.

A continuing concern of practitioners of therapies that are considering the transition from VSR to SSR is how much it will cost them. The cost of maintaining any regulatory body, whether voluntary or statutory, is borne by the members through annual subscription fees. Currently this may be as much as £1000 each year to remain on the chiropractors' register.

Another concern for CAM therapists is whether their current qualifications are sufficient to gain entry to a statutory register. Once a statutory scheme is established, a relevant qualification from an approved training institution secures entry to the statutory register. However, when a statutory register is created for the first time, transitional arrangements have to be negotiated in order to determine who should be admitted to the initial register of members. In making the transition from voluntary to statutory status, all existing therapists have to satisfy their new statutory council that they provide safe and competent treatment. Fitness to practise also requires practitioners to demonstrate that they are in good physical and mental health. In short, practitioners have to demonstrate competence in various ways required of them by the regulatory body. The establishment of the osteopaths register required therapists to prepare an extensive Professional Practice Portfolio and, for some practitioners, there were interviews and site visits to their place of practice.

A statutory scheme usually involves practitioners undertaking appropriate CPD. In CAM therapies, the costs of keeping up to date in this way are borne directly by individual practitioners. A voluntary regulatory body, on the other hand, may strongly encourage its members to keep their professional skills up to date but probably lacks the power to enforce this requirement.

For practitioners who have had many successful years in practice, or those nearing retirement, the thought of meeting these additional regulatory requirements may be unappealing.

It is worth reflecting that some of the objections to regulation demonstrate a high level of self-interest. Public safety should be the paramount concern for any health care practitioner. Clearly, regulation is more burdensome than no regulation, but practitioners are aware that not all therapists are conscientious and practise in a safe way. Regulation that weeds out dangerous or poorly performing practitioners should be welcomed.

For CAM users

It is easy to say that better regulation ensures a better standard of care for CAM users but that link is not necessarily measurable. Poor professional performance and misconduct exist even within highly regulated professions such as medicine and nursing. External regulation is not a cure-all. Practitioners are individually accountable for their actions, whatever form of regulation they are subject to. However, the more effective the regulation, the more likely it is that there are effective means of redress if something does go wrong.

In fact, the area where CAM users are most likely to benefit from better regulation is not necessarily fitness to practise but in terms of therapeutic developments. The capacity for research within a therapy requires a highly developed professional infrastructure. This is more achievable in a therapy with established, externally validated educational procedures, high levels of pre- and postgraduate training, and institutional links with other health care professions. These hallmarks are far more likely to be found in a highly regulated therapy.

For the medical profession

Because CAM is no longer considered a marginal aspect of health care delivery, some orthodox doctors are increasingly keen to ensure that 'their' patients are adequately protected from what they see as bogus or inadequately qualified practitioners. Given the intense hostility displayed by some sectors of the orthodox medical profession towards CAM in the past (see, for example, British Medical Association, 1986), these calls for tighter regulation might be motivated by bias and medical protectionism. Yet, as Stone and Matthews argue, the regulatory inconsistency between orthodox and non-orthodox medicine is untenable:

> [T]he existing discrepancy between an intensely regulated orthodox profession and the formally unregulated position of most complementary therapies will become increasingly difficult to justify. Mainstream medicine is, today, one of the most highly regulated of all social and economic activities. With this firmly in mind, and at a time when so great an emphasis is being placed on consumer rights in health care, on what basis are we able to defend a situation in which so much of complementary medicine remains apparently unregulated? On the face of it, it is not only illogical, but hazardous.
>
> (Stone and Matthews, 1996, p. 5)

Orthodox doctors are concerned that the lack of 'scientific' evidence supporting many CAM therapies means that CAM users may be exposed to an unacceptable level of risk. It is even argued that, in the absence of such evidence, users cannot give informed consent to CAM procedures (Ernst, 1996).

ACTIVITY   HOW DO YOU KNOW IT WILL WORK?

Allow 10 minutes

Think back again to when you consulted a CAM therapist. Did you have any form of treatment? If so, did you comply with the treatment because you had 'scientific' evidence that it would work? If you have never consulted a CAM therapist, how important would it be to you to see such evidence before having treatment?

Comment

Most users seem untroubled by the lack of 'scientific' evidence and consult CAM therapists because the therapy seems to work for them. After all, if it does not work they will not return for more. However, safety is another matter. The evidence necessary to demonstrate safety is discussed in Chapter 7.

The medical profession's insistence that CAM improves its evidence base may partly be a manifestation of the medical profession's exasperation with some CAM therapists' defiantly anti-scientific stance. It is understandable that doctors perceive the lack of evidence base in CAM to be unacceptable when there is an increasing insistence that they themselves work in an evidence-based way.

Medical attitudes towards CAM have changed significantly since the British Medical Association's report *Alternative Therapies* (BMA, 1986). The resolutely hostile attitude that once characterised the official position of orthodox medicine to non-conventional therapies has mellowed since then. There are encouraging signs of a greater spirit of tolerance and co-operation, fostered no doubt by a recognition of political realities as well as by a genuine change of attitude. Increasing numbers of doctors use CAM in their work or refer their patients to CAM therapists. The desire for better regulation and evidence of efficacy can be seen as part of a genuine desire for doctors to feel confident about incorporating CAM into people's treatment if it will be of benefit. They argue that when CAM treatment goes wrong, they have to pick up the pieces. They say people may be harmed in two ways:

1   where a therapy is directly harmful if practised by an untrained or incompetent practitioner

2   if the patient is prevented from seeking appropriate orthodox care which could provide a more effective cure, the implication being that harm may be a consequence of serious medical problems being undetected or ignored (BMA, 1993).

Stone and Matthews (1996) argue that the second type of harm is prompted more by political considerations and is not supported by evidence that this is happening on a wide scale. They also point out that, while theoretically a legal action could be based on the first sort of harm, it is almost impossible in the second situation, since the choice to accept or reject medical advice or treatment lies within the realm of patient choice.

For NHS and other policy makers

CAM professions need to have a cohesive and strong political voice to be included in policy debates at the highest levels of the NHS. In keeping with the evidence-based approach that now underpins other health professions, CAM therapies will be required to have a track record of research and audit and must be able to show that their therapy is both safe and efficacious. As discussed in Section 3.4, this is more achievable for a statutorily regulated profession than for a voluntarily regulated profession.

Although integration of CAM and orthodox medicine in the NHS does not necessarily depend on the transition of CAM therapies from VSR to SSR, the following points can be realistically inferred from the integration debates.

1 NHS purchasers of CAM services will require the strongest reassurance about the competence of CAM practitioners. This is likely to incline them towards contracting with statutorily regulated professionals.

2 Integration will be into an increasingly evidence-based culture, requiring a more highly developed research base.

3 CAM will be integrated into an already cash-starved NHS and will require evidence of cost-effectiveness as well as efficacy.

4 CAM therapies will have an improved chance of negotiating their place in the 'New NHS' if they come together under a single regulatory authority for each profession. The lack of professional cohesion makes it difficult for a purchaser to know who to negotiate with at a profession-wide level.

3.6 Conclusion

This chapter discussed the issues and debates concerning the regulation of complementary and alternative medicine in the UK. Many people believe that a single professional register of CAM therapists is desirable, to allow potential users and policy makers to determine who is and who is not appropriately qualified. A single professional register has the potential to minimise confusion, but internal disputes within each modality often seem to mitigate against this outcome. Therapies which could cause direct, physical harm would appear to be most in need of vigorous, external regulation. Even therapies which seem to confer no obvious benefit can, in the wrong hands, potentially harm users and therefore require some form of regulation.

Regulation may give an air of respectability to a particular therapy and thereby be a means of enhancing public respect and status. However, in the long run this may be better earned by therapists from different modalities consistently demonstrating high standards of practice and ethical awareness. Statutory regulation is certainly more likely to ensure high uniform standards of training and practice for each type of therapy. Statutory regulation is more effective than voluntary self-regulation, although it remains to be seen what would happen if a significant number of professionals refused to join a statutory register. Statutory regulation may represent a significant cost for members of a CAM profession: the smaller the profession, potentially the higher the costs that will have to be shared.

Although research and development is much harder when there is a lack of professional cohesion and fragmentation, statutory regulation may lead to a loss of diversity within a profession and a loss of innovative or radical features. Since the late 1990s there has been a movement both towards increased regulation of CAM and for the regulatory bodies themselves to be under surveillance, to ensure that they are keeping up the standards and consistency within their profession.

KEY POINTS

- There is a general movement towards increased surveillance, regulation and control of people who offer therapies and all forms of health care.
- This increased regulatory effort is partly a reaction to the serious misconduct of some individuals and institutions and follows the recommendations of various committees set up to study these incidents.
- CAM organisations will be under increasing pressure to scrutinise the activities of their therapists, whether through voluntary or statutory regulation.
- Clear guidelines and principles have been established to help determine how the health sector should be regulated.
- In a scheme of voluntary regulation, the regulatory body may have only limited powers to control the therapists on their register. Statutory regulation, however, may not be appropriate for all CAM therapies.
- Although a single regulatory body seems ideal for each CAM therapy, internal differences within some modalities have made it impossible to achieve that aim.

References

Allsop, J. and Mulcahy, L. (1996) *Regulating Medical Work: Formal and Informal Controls*, Buckingham, Open University Press.

Allsop, J. and Saks, M. (eds) (2002) *Regulating the Health Professions*, London, Sage Publications.

Better Regulation Task Force (2000) *Alternatives to State Regulation*, London, The Cabinet Office.

British Medical Association (1986) *Report of the Board of Science: Alternative Therapy*, London, BMA.

British Medical Association (1993) *Complementary Medicine: New Approaches to Good Practice*, London, BMA.

Cohen, M. (1998) *Complementary and Alternative Medicine: Legal Boundaries and Regulatory Perspectives*, Baltimore, MD, Johns Hopkins University Press.

Commission for Alternative Systems of Medicine (1981) *Alternative Medicine in the Netherlands*, The Hague, Staatsuitgeverij.

Department of Health (1997) *The New NHS: Modern, Dependable*, London, HMSO.

Department of Health (2001a) *Modernising Regulation in the Health Professions*, London, The Stationery Office.

Department of Health (2001b) *Meeting the Challenge: A Strategy for the Allied Health Professions*, London, The Stationery Office.

Department of Health (2001c) *Modernising Regulation: The New Health Professions Council*, London, Department of Health.

Department of Health (2001d) *Government Response to the House of Lords Select Committee on Science and Technology's Report on Complementary and Alternative Medicine*, CM 5124, London, DoH. Available online at: www.archive.official-documents.co.uk/document/cm51/5124/5124.pdf [accessed 2 October 2004].

Ernst, E. (1996) 'The ethics of complementary medicine', *Journal of Medical Ethics*, Vol. 22, pp. 197–8.

House of Lords (2000) Sixth Report of the House of Lords Committee on Science and Technology, *Complementary and Alternative Medicine*, London, The Stationery Office. Available online at: www.parliament.the-stationery-office.co.UK/pa/ldl99900/1dselect/idstech/123/12301.htm [accessed 2 October 2004].

JM Consulting (1998) *The Regulation of Nurses, Midwives and Health Visitors: Report on a Review of the Nurses, Midwives and Health Visitors Act 1997*, Bristol, JM Consulting Ltd.

Kennedy, I. (2001) *Learning from Bristol: The Report of the Public Inquiry into Children's Surgery at the Bristol Royal Infirmary 1984–1995*, Cm 5207 (1), London, The Stationery Office. Available online at: www.bristol-inquiry.org.uk/final_report/ [accessed 2 October 2004].

Mills, S. (2001) 'Regulation in complementary and alternative medicine', *British Medical Journal*, Vol. 322, pp. 158–60.

Moran, M. and Wood, B. (1993) *States, Regulation and the Medical Profession*, Buckingham, Open University Press.

Price, D. (2002) 'Legal aspects of the regulation of the health professions', in Allsop and Saks, pp. 47–61.

Redfern, M. (2001) *Royal Liverpool Children's Inquiry*, London, House of Commons. Available online at: www.rlcinquiry.org.uk/download/chap1.pdf [accessed 2 October 2004].

Stone, J. (1996) Editorial: 'Regulating complementary medicine: standards not status', *British Medical Journal*, Vol. 312, pp. 1492–3.

Stone, J. and Matthews, J. (1995) 'The effective regulation of complementary medicine', *Complementary Therapies in Medicine*, Vol. 3, pp. 175–8.

Stone, J. and Matthews, J. (1996) *Complementary Medicine and the Law*, Oxford, Oxford University Press.

White, C. (2004) 'Regulatory body proposed for acupuncturists and herbalists', *British Medical Journal*, Vol. 328, p. 604.

Chapter 4 Political power and professionalisation

Mike Saks and Geraldine Lee-Treweek

Contents

AIMS

- To critically analyse the features of a profession and relate them to the health care professions.
- To debate the advantages and disadvantages of the professionalisation of CAM for practitioners, users and orthodox medical professionals.

4.1 Introduction

In the UK, the notion of being 'professional' has many different connotations in everyday language – from a job well done to paid work, as distinct from work done by amateurs. In academic terms, the concept of a 'profession' generally refers to a more powerful, higher-ranking and financially better-rewarded occupation, which, among other features, can engage in self-regulation – typically with the blessing of the state. Such occupations range from architects and social workers to doctors and lawyers, the latter two frequently being seen as classic professions. In this chapter 'professions' in the academic sense and the associated notion of 'professionalisation' – which is the process by which an occupation becomes a profession – are discussed with reference to different theoretical approaches drawn from the social sciences.

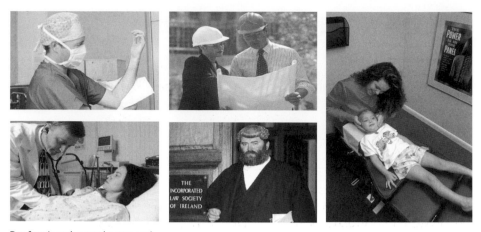

Professional people at work

The definitions of professions based on these approaches span from those centred on a more positive view of such groups to those with a more jaundiced perspective.

First, this chapter examines the range of theoretical approaches on offer and, using examples from the health field, makes the case for adopting a particular approach to the professions. This is a politicised view of professions in so far as it infers that these groups use political power to advance their own interests against their rivals. This approach is then applied, first, to the general development of medicine and the allied health professions and, second, to the more recent professionalisation of aspects of CAM in the UK. Finally, the future of professionalisation is considered, alongside the advantages and disadvantages of professionalisation. These are examined with particular reference to the various CAM stakeholders – the public, orthodox health professions and CAM practitioners themselves.

4.2 Perspectives on professions and professionalisation

The nature of a profession – and hence the process of professionalisation – has been the subject of much disagreement in the social sciences. Before exploring the different social science perspectives, spend a few minutes reflecting on your own taken-for-granted notions of the concept of 'profession'.

ACTIVITY   WHAT IS A PROFESSIONAL?

Allow 10 minutes

How would you define the term 'professional'? Look at the phrases listed below. What aspect of professions and professionalisation do they convey?

Professional conduct	A professional job	A real pro
Professionally qualified	The caring professions	Turning professional

Comment

Your definition may include aspects of the notion of being a 'professional' mentioned in the introduction to this chapter. Certainly the phrases 'a professional job' and 'a real pro' give a sense of a job well done and not amateurish. Similarly, 'turning professional' involves a change in status from amateur to paid professional mainly in the area of sport. Being professionally qualified and professional conduct are elements of 'the professions' which can engage in self-regulation, such as doctors and lawyers. How did the notion of the caring professions fit with your definition? It seems to convey a degree of altruism with the public good as the main motivating force. This raises the question of whether professions and professionalisation are a positive or a negative force in society – a question that has exercised social scientists' minds about professions.

The rest of this section describes several social science theories, which have very different ideas about the role of 'a profession' and the question of whether it represents a positive or a negative force in society, especially in relation to its responsibilities to the general public.

Professions: a positive or a negative force in society?

Early work in the sociology of professions, particularly in health work, was based on the **functionalist** approach of Talcott Parsons (1951). Advocates of this approach believed that the leading professions such as medicine and law were distinguished from other occupations by the positive and significant part they played in society (Millerson, 1964). Functionalist authors focused on the elements of a profession that they believed were of functional significance for the wider society and/or their individual clients – such as their specialist knowledge. These theorists can be said to have a positive attitude to professions, seeing them as necessary groups contributing to the benefit of society. By using their distinctive expertise non-exploitatively for the public good, they earned their privileged financial and social status (Goode, 1960; Barber, 1963). Their position is explained in Box 4.1 (overleaf).

professional groups because it challenges the rationality of scientific knowledge. Foucault (1980) was interested in the relationship between knowledge and power. He argued that professions such as medicine and the law could exercise power and control because they defined and determined what counts as knowledge in a particular field. Foucault called these bodies of knowledge 'discourses'. Legal discourses relate to crime, punishment and legal practice but they also define what can be considered a legal matter, so they in fact determine the territory that is considered to be the prerogative of the legal profession and thus the basis of its power. Foucault argued that these discourses were based on the 'interests' of different groups and he was concerned with how one set of discourses becomes dominant. Biomedicine is a prime example of the way in which medical knowledge has been constructed and defined to protect the interests of the medical profession and to effect social closure, where one group takes control of the knowledge territory. This determines not only who can and cannot enter the profession but also what the public need in order to be healthy. The Foucaldian approach to dentistry is described in Box 4.3.

BOX 4.3   THE FOUCALDIAN APPROACH TO THE HEALTH PROFESSIONS

Sarah Nettleton (1992) illustrates the **Foucaldian approach** to the health professions by applying this perspective to dentistry. Her analysis considers the historical relationship between dental power and dental knowledge in the UK. Relating Foucault's ideas on power and knowledge to the mouth and teeth and the profession of dentistry, she concludes that the rise of the dental profession was not based primarily on establishing the most effective and appropriate treatment in this field. The development and power of dentistry is based on its ability to convince others of the need to monitor the mouth and teeth. In convincing others, especially the state, of this the profession secures for itself a position of power. As she says: 'The discipline of dentistry did not simply emerge because of treatment needs or because of the demands for legislation to ensure enclosure of the profession, but more through the techniques of public health which served to ensure policing of mouths and the monitoring of teeth' (Nettleton, 1992, p. 127).

Another approach which takes a much less positive view than the functionalist perspective is the **neo-Weberian approach**. This has drawn on and developed the work of the German sociologist Max Weber (1864–1920), who originally outlined the concept of exclusionary closure centred on market control (Weber, 1968, first published 1922). The neo-Weberian approach defines professions simply in terms of the state-supported legal monopoly that they hold in the market, limiting access to the profession to a restricted group whose names appear on a register (Parkin, 1979). Freidson (1983) claims that this 'market shelter' protects the profession from outsiders. It also links to concepts of professionalism based on occupational control over both the organisation of work and definitions of client needs (as exemplified by Freidson, 1970; Johnson, 1972). The analysis of the role of self-interests in defending and/or enhancing the monopolistic position of professions is central to neo-Weberian studies, which usually focus on conflicts of interest involving professional and other occupational groups – not least including medicine and CAM (Larkin, 1995).

Everyday use of the terms 'professional' and 'professionalisation' centres on distinctions between the amateur and the paid professional, the highly qualified and the unqualified. Sociological approaches have attempted a more critical analysis of professions, focusing very much on their potential as a positive or a negative force in society. This has created a great deal of debate and controversy. The narrative running through the analysis of different sociological perspectives sets out with a rather optimistic, benign functionalist view of professions being of benefit to wider society. This view is based on their having certain traits (such as codes of ethics, expertise and knowledge) which are in the public interest. The interactionist view sounds warning bells about accepting this version of reality uncritically. The Marxist and Foucaldian approaches go much further in arguing for a decidedly negative analysis of professions. In the Marxist account they are regarded as oppressive organs of the capitalist enterprise. In the Foucaldian account the use of knowledge to maintain their power and control is seen as far from benign. The neo-Weberian analysis is attractive in that it allows for a more pragmatic approach, acknowledging the role of self-interest of professions but not going so far as to construe this as malevolent or necessarily against the public interest.

So, the neo-Weberian approach offers significant advantages over other perspectives on professions. It is no longer necessary automatically to see professional groups in a positive light as many functionalist writers have done. The neo-Weberian perspective also considers the structural and historical dimensions of professions and professionalisation at a wider sociopolitical level. In this light, it is not surprising that social scientists use the neo-Weberian approach so widely to examine professions in the UK.

ACTIVITY SELF-INTEREST OR PUBLIC INTEREST?

Allow 20 minutes

Draw up a balance sheet between self-interest and public interest of professional status based on your reading of this chapter so far, and drawing on the arguments for statutory state regulation required for professional status that were discussed in Chapter 3.

Comment

Certainly the arguments for self-interest are strong: the protection of title and function and market protection give security, status and income. However, on the other side of the balance sheet, statutory state regulation aims to protect the public from fraud and to ensure a well qualified, knowledgeable profession that operates with an ethical code of conduct. These issues are considered in more detail in the next section, specifically in the context of the health professions.

4.3 The development of the medical and allied professions

Berlant (1975) applied a neo-Weberian analysis to the rise of the medical profession in both the UK and the USA. He argues that the success of doctors in gaining state underwriting for their privileged position was a result of both their tactics and the socioeconomic conditions that existed in a competitive marketplace. The establishment of a unified medical profession in the UK through the Medical Registration Act 1858 centred on the formation of the General Medical Council. As described in Chapter 3, this body, dominated by doctors, held a register of practitioners and provided the basis for the self-regulation of the profession, in matters ranging from discipline to education. According to Berlant, a key reason for the success of medicine in establishing and maintaining the legally underwritten social closure of the profession against outsiders was the skilful way in which it managed to side-step 19th-century attacks on the profession for holding a monopoly over practice. One way in which it did this was to allow competitors to continue to practise under the Common Law.

Parry and Parry (1977) argue that the monopoly that was established in the UK, in which the title 'medical doctor' was restricted to those on the register, led to the collective upward social mobility of the medical profession. In this regard, increasing market control drove up the overall income, status and power of its members. This control and the associated privileges rose still further with the passing of the National Health Insurance Act 1911 and the National Health Service Act 1946. This legislation not only expanded the amount of state-funded medical practice in which qualified doctors could exclusively engage but also enhanced the legitimacy and public image of the profession as a whole.

Saks (1996) observes that the strength of professionalised medicine also derived from the growing coherence of the knowledge base of its members. This was increasingly focused on the development of the 'scientific' biomedical paradigm. Another aspect of its strength up to the mid-20th century was its success in sidelining its CAM rivals through the process of medical professionalisation. This took many forms, including:

■ attacks on CAM practitioners in the mainstream medical journals for being 'unscientific' and for robbing patients of their money
■ the establishment of a professional code of ethics limiting collaboration with non-medically qualified CAM practitioners, under threat of disciplinary action
■ restrictions on the career prospects of orthodox medical practitioners who practised or sympathised with CAM
■ blocking attempts by groups of CAM practitioners such as herbalists and osteopaths to gain professional recognition.

It is debatable whether these tactics were in the public interest. Functionalist writers such as Wallis and Morley (1976) tend to see the professionalisation of medicine, and the consequent marginalisation of CAM, as a rational step enabling patients, through the revolution in medical treatment, to cope better with disease and be protected from exploitation. It is easy to see how this view of medicine as a selfless and caring profession precludes a more critical view of this occupational group. However, what cannot be disputed from a neo-Weberian, interests-based viewpoint is the fact that medically qualified practitioners had an interest in gaining and sustaining their professional standing – not least by belittling CAM practitioners whenever the opportunity arose.

The success of the medical profession in the UK was ultimately sealed by such factors as political support from the developing pharmaceutical industry and divisions in the ranks of CAM practitioners themselves (Saks, 1996). However, most fundamental to the professionalisation of medicine was the backing of the state. This also enabled the medical profession at a later stage to subordinate or limit the authority of potential rivals in the health field, through their incorporation into orthodox health care but under the power and direction of medicine. In these cases, incorporation typically involved ongoing, interest-based fighting over territory, in which the dominant medical profession that had already accomplished social closure was greatly advantaged. From this standpoint, medicine could use this power to ensure that the professionalisation of other health groups took place in the most favourable manner with respect to its own interests – through either subordination or limitation (Saks, 2003).

Turner (1995) identifies the following categories of professionalisation of the allied health professions.

1 **Subordination:** where the profession takes on tasks delegated by doctors.
2 **Limitation:** where the operation of a profession is limited to a particular therapeutic method or part of the body.

ACTIVITY   MAINTAINING MEDICAL DOMINANCE

Allow 15 minutes

Which occupational groups fall into the two categories of subordination and limitation in the UK?

Comment

Subordinated professional groups in the UK include those such as midwives and nurses, founded through the Midwives Act 1902 and the Nursing Registration Act 1919 respectively, and occupations such as chiropodists, dieticians, physiotherapists and radiographers, established through the Professions Supplementary to Medicine Act 1960. Limited professional groups are best exemplified by pharmacists established by the Pharmacy Acts in the 1850s and 1860s, dentists by the Dentists Act 1878 and opticians through the Opticians Act 1958. This legislation ultimately enabled all these groups to found their own governing councils, from the General Nursing Council and the Council of the Professions Supplementary to Medicine to the General Dental Council and the General Optical Council (see, for example, Larkin, 1983; Stacey, 1988). These councils were distinguished by the fact that they had an overwhelming majority of professional members and functioned in a complementary way to the General Medical Council (Stacey, 1992).

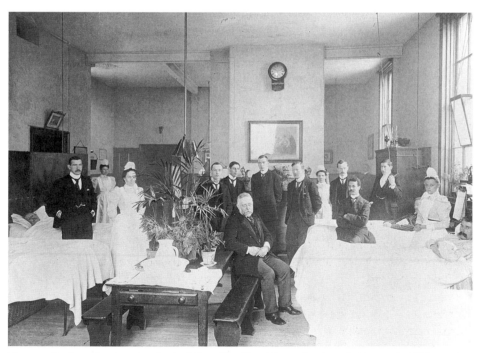

The medical profession dominated the allied health professions in the early 20th century

Given the tradition of medical dominance, it is not surprising that the allied health professions are often referred to as **semi-professions**. With a neo-Weberian perspective, Parkin (1979) believes that many of the semi-professions, such as nursing and teaching, are increasingly in a position of 'dual closure' in which – having failed to win the full professional standing of medicine – they contain elements of both exclusionary closure based on credentialism and trade unionism linked to organised labour. In other words, while kept out of the ranks of top professions, these groups exclude others by insisting on such issues as stringent professional qualifications for members. At the same time, they use trade union tactics to defend their interests. The semi-professional standing of such groups was reinforced by being predominantly female in contrast to the exclusive male origins of the medical profession. This was also a material factor in the subjugated way in which they developed in a patriarchal society (Witz, 1992).

Jones (1994) maintains that the sociology of the professions had in general overlooked the question of gender relationships. She argues that feminist theory provided a much richer analysis of gendered occupations in health work:

> In particular, it draws attention to the fact that the professionalisation of medicine represented not just a triumph of a middle class occupational group but the gendering of power and privilege within health work. It was the institutionalisation of male dominance that ensured, in some form, female subordination.
>
> (Jones, 1994, p. 432)

In contrast, functionalist writers such as Etzioni (1969) believe that the lower position of occupational groups like nurses in the professional pecking order is because they intrinsically need less expertise and training to carry out their role. However, as indicated above, from a neo-Weberian standpoint, it is difficult not to view the secondary standing of the allied health professions in relation to medicine primarily in terms of interest-group politics based on ongoing medical dominance. That said, the standing of the more established health professions is now being radically challenged, as they have been under increasing attack in the UK since the mid-20th century.

The growing challenge to the health professions from the 1960s and 1970s onwards largely derived from consumer lobbies and government attempts to exert more control over doctors. This led the Conservative government to try to diminish the power of the health professions from the late 1970s onwards, through such measures as the Griffiths reforms in 1983, which were aimed at increasing independent management of the National Health Service (NHS); the introduction of the Patient's Charter in 1991; and the subsequent establishment of the purchaser–provider split to reduce professional influence over decision making (Saks, 2003). At first it appeared that the power of the medical and other professions would block significant change (Elston, 1991). However, in the early 1990s general practitioners increased their power within the medical profession at the expense of hospital specialists, with growing state support for primary care (Allsop, 1995). Moreover, from the late 1990s the agenda of health professional reform was even more proactively carried forward by the Labour government, in the wake of increasing political concern about professions abusing their self-regulating powers.

In the light of cases of abuse of professional powers (such as Harold Shipman and others outlined in Chapter 3) and the growing political emphasis on protecting the public, the government has closely scrutinised the health professions and their governing councils. This led to a wide range of reforms. The General Medical Council, for example, introduced several changes to increase public confidence, such as a scheme to reaccredit practising doctors, tightening up fitness-to-practise procedures and substantially increasing the proportion of its lay members (Allsop, 2002). At the same time, the United Kingdom Central Council and the English National Board for Nursing, Midwifery and Health Visiting – which replaced the original General Nursing Council – have now become the more accountable and transparent Nursing and Midwifery Council. This has an even split between its lay and professional members, thereby increasing public involvement in professional affairs (Davies, 2002). The Council for the Professions Supplementary to Medicine has also been transformed into the streamlined Health Professions Council, with an enhanced lay membership and the removal of the historic cap on the number of constituent professions registered with it (Larkin, 2002). In addition, the government recently established the innovatory Council for Healthcare Regulatory Excellence (CHRE), to oversee regulatory issues across the health professions (Allsop and Saks, 2002).

ACTIVITY   QUESTIONING PROFESSIONS

Allow 20 minutes

Do you think that there is a more critical view now of the concepts of professions and professionalisation, in the light of the recent government desire to reform the health professions? Are professions still regarded with reverence or are questions raised about how they operate in practice?

Comment

Your response probably depends on your experiences of health professionals. You may be a health professional yourself. In general, older people still maintain much respect for 'the doctor' but, as the generation that experienced life before the NHS dies, that reverence may disappear. Certainly, doctors are not regarded with awe but they are still high on the list of respected professions. However, with greater awareness of health issues and access to medical knowledge on the internet, lay people are much more inclined to question their doctors' diagnosis and treatment.

4.4   The professionalisation of CAM

Section 4.3 provides a useful context for understanding the recent professionalisation of some forms of CAM in the UK. As described earlier in this chapter, CAM was marginalised from the 19th century onwards as a result of the professionalisation of medicine. The legal framework underpinning medical professionalisation created a large group of disenfranchised outsiders, which contrasted with the relatively open, pluralistic field that had previously existed. Although they could continue to practise under the Common Law, these CAM outsiders were in turn subject to further attack as the medical profession sought to preserve and extend its own interests in establishing its monopoly (Saks, 1999).

However, despite the negative implications of professionalisation for their own position, groups of CAM practitioners also had an interest in gaining professional standing from the viewpoint of income, status and power. None the less, despite the professionalisation of a range of allied health professions on terms favourable to orthodox medicine, attempts by CAM practitioners to gain their own professional status foundered at the hands of the strong medical–ministry alliance that existed up to the late 20th century. This is well illustrated by the case of osteopaths, who unsuccessfully lobbied to gain professional standing as early as the 1920s and 1930s (see Box 4.4). They were primarily thwarted by the power and interests of the medical establishment, supported by the expanding pharmaceutical industry, which generally saw CAM as a direct commercial challenge (Saks, 1996).

BOX 4.4   OSTEOPATHY IN THE 1920s AND 1930s: A CASE OF THWARTED PROFESSIONALISATION

Larkin (1992) documents how claims for the state registration of osteopathy as a profession escalated in the 1920s and 1930s, with the backing of some Members of Parliament. However, there was great resistance from the medical profession. As Larkin notes, in 1925 the *British Medical Journal* argued that osteopaths were encroaching on medicine because they were under threat from the chiropractors and were seeking to enter medical practice by the back door. Since they held fundamentally conflicting theories of medicine, the challenging claims from osteopathic competitors were treated with derision. The theory that conditions such as colds, gout and measles could be due to small spinal irregularities, for example, were dismissed as 'far-fetched and fanciful' and 'decidedly dangerous' when applied to grave diseases such as typhoid fever and diphtheria. Given the threat to medical interests and the strength of the medical–ministry alliance, it is not surprising that several subsequent Bills aimed at gaining independent osteopathic registration in the 1930s were blocked after opposition by the medical profession.

The position changed in the 1960s and 1970s with increasing public demand for mainstream CAM therapies from acupuncture to homeopathy, which was linked to the emerging medical counter-culture. This gave rise to political lobbies in favour of the fast-growing number of non-medically qualified CAM practitioners – not least through HRH Prince Charles and the all-party Parliamentary Group for Alternative and Complementary Medicine (Saks, 2002). In these circumstances, incorporation on the appropriate terms rather than the outright rejection of CAM became the order of the day for the medical profession. The removal of ethical barriers to such collaboration by the General Medical Council (GMC) from the mid-1970s and the British Medical Association (BMA) by the late 1980s facilitated an incorporationist strategy. By the early 1990s, the interest-based benefits to most orthodox medical practitioners in collaborating with CAM therapists with appropriately certified credentials – including medical subjects such as physiology and anatomy – had become apparent (BMA, 1993).

Osteopathy has now at last gained the formal standing of a profession with a statutory register through a field-breaking private member's Bill. Although there have been substantial internal rifts historically in this area (Fulder, 1996), there was sufficient agreement for the Osteopaths Act to be passed in 1993. The well-regarded educational framework for osteopathy, together with its wider political backing, also helped the Act to be passed. The legislation gives the newly formed General Osteopathic Council such tasks as holding a register of practitioners, protecting titles, engaging in the self-regulation of peers, and maintaining relevant ethical and educational standards (Saks, 2002).

However, this did not resolve the problem of the disunity of CAM therapists in progressing the professionalisation agenda. This was an issue in the 1980s when the Conservative government sought a unified approach from all CAM therapies before proceeding with legislation on professional regulation (Sharma, 1995). But this was never going to be practically realised in view of the deep-seated divisions within CAM at this stage (Fulder, 1996), despite organisational efforts to increase unity through the Institute for Complementary Medicine, the Council for Complementary and Alternative Medicine, and the British Complementary Medical Association. Fortunately, by the early 1990s the government had ruled that particular forms of CAM should present their own case for professionalisation in the health arena. This improved the chances of non-medical practitioners of individual CAM therapies in their search for professional recognition (Cant and Sharma, 1999).

Before further charting the outcome of this search, note that in terms of professionalisation many orthodox health professionals – from general practitioners to nurses and physiotherapists – now use CAM therapies (Saks, 2001). However, members of medical bodies such as the British Medical Acupuncture Society and the Faculty of Homoeopathy have frequently done so in a manner more compatible with the biomedical paradigm than the traditional theories associated with many CAM practices. They have also formed an important part of the resistance to the professionalisation of CAM outsiders. From the viewpoint of medical self-interests, such CAM groups can be seen as rivals who increasingly compete for paying clients in the private sector and whose philosophies often directly challenge their biomedical knowledge. Although, arguably, there are public health gains from adopting a negative stance towards less convincing types of CAM, such medical interests in augmenting income, status and power appear to have been central to the process of ongoing exclusion (Saks, 1995).

Despite such pockets of continuing resistance, some CAM areas are becoming professionalised, even though this has varied greatly in specific CAM therapies in the UK. The least professionalised therapies typically are those used largely on a self-help basis and relying on a limited knowledge base, such as crystal therapy. Although more generally accepted, CAM therapies such as aromatherapy and reflexology have also not gone far down the path of professionalisation. While these therapies have thousands of practitioners, their training is typically fairly short, and there is a broad range of educational establishments and associations (Cant and Sharma, 1995). Admittedly this is changing, as their training schools and organisations increasingly adopt similar standards, but there is still a long way to go compared with other CAM practices.

ACTIVITY   DIFFERENT TYPES OF EDUCATION AND TRAINING

Allow 15 minutes

Which factors in the education and training of CAM practitioners discussed in Chapter 2 made it difficult to present a unified profession?

Comment

You may recall the debate from Cant's work on the difference between informal 'charismatic' teaching and more formal academic methods. Some modalities seemed more suited to the charismatic way, yet others adopted the academic way with various forms of accreditation. Similarly, there was a debate about the suitability of apprenticeships as opposed to academic qualifications. The problem of getting agreement on a core curriculum also made it difficult for some modalities to present themselves as a unified profession.

Some groups of CAM practitioners have progressed much further in establishing unified mechanisms for voluntary self-regulation – without as yet gaining the statutory regulation that underpins the registration arrangements for the established health professions. For instance, the Council for Acupuncture was established on a voluntary basis in 1980 by several previously divided acupuncture associations (see Box 4.5 overleaf). The Council was initially rooted in a common code of discipline, education and ethics. It subsequently developed in the late 1980s with the emergence of the British Acupuncture Accreditation Board, which lays down minimum educational standards, and the British Acupuncture Council, which registers practitioners (Saks, 1995).

> ### BOX 4.5   VOLUNTARY SELF-REGULATION AS A STEP TOWARDS PROFESSIONALISATION: THE CASE OF ACUPUNCTURE
>
> Saks (2002) suggests that establishing a coherent system of voluntary self-regulation is no easy task given the divisions within CAM. This is highlighted by the case of acupuncture, where the formation of the Council for Acupuncture in 1980 brought together the following previously disparate non-medical organisations of practitioners:
>
> - the British Acupuncture Association and Register
> - the Chung San Acupuncture Society
> - the International Register of Oriental Medicine
> - the Register of Traditional Chinese Medicine
> - the Traditional Acupuncture Society.
>
> Such unifying work is extremely important politically in the professionalising process. Acupuncture has now reached the point where it can launch a credible bid for statutory regulation – especially given the potential hazards that this invasive therapy poses to the public that enable it to draw on protectionist ideologies.

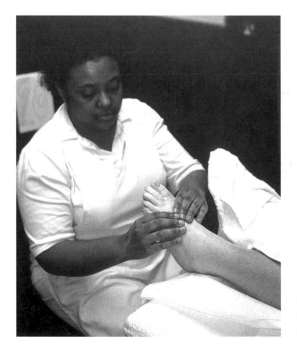

Some complementary and alternative therapies are not yet professionalised

There have been similar developments in terms of voluntary self-regulation elsewhere, not least in homeopathy where the Society of Homoeopaths is the major body representing non-medically qualified practitioners. Since its formation in 1981, the Society has established a self-administered register and code of ethics. While this sphere of CAM is not at present as unified as acupuncture, the Society of Homoeopaths formally accredits training at an increasing number of homeopathic colleges. Within these colleges a systematic body of expertise has emerged, based on a model of three-year, full-time education (Cant and Sharma, 1996). However, as in the case of acupuncture, a legally underwritten position of exclusionary closure has yet to be achieved. The situation with homeopathy is developed further in Chapter 5.

ACTIVITY   THE MARK OF A PROFESSION

Allow 15 minutes

Examine the advertisements for different CAM modalities in Figure 4.1. How do they convey a sense of professionalism? How reassuring do you find them?

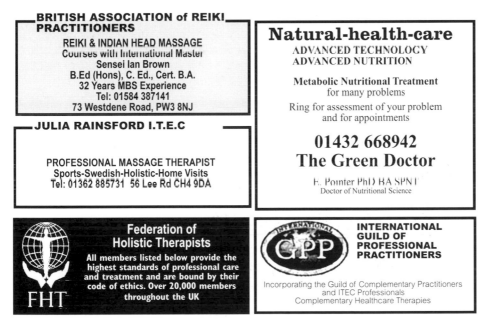

Figure 4.1   Advertisements for CAM therapists

Comment

Some have formed a federation and others a guild of practitioners, which implies a code of ethical conduct. Others have letters after their names, indicating relevant qualifications. Unless the letters mean something to you, it is hard to be reassured about how competent the practitioners are. However, it should be possible to check up on the qualifications and to verify the credibility of the register.

The legislation underpinning osteopathy was followed by the Chiropractors Act 1994, which established a similar type of state regulation for chiropractors, centred on the General Chiropractic Council (Cant and Sharma, 1995). However, while this Act has improved the market position and enhanced the legitimacy of chiropractic in the UK – in much the same way as for osteopathy – there are limitations. Neither of these practices has privileged access to funding in the state health service in contrast to the orthodox health professions, even though the exclusionary self-regulatory model in both cases is drawn from medicine (Saks, 1999). From a neo-Weberian market perspective, chiropractors and osteopaths are therefore still at a competitive disadvantage from the viewpoint of professionalisation.

However, the growing strength of the position of such therapists in the professional fold raises other concerns because it draws further attention to potential gender discrimination issues in health professionalisation in the UK. Note that, although most practitioners in CAM are women, the first CAM groups to gain statutory regulation – chiropractic and osteopathy – are male-dominated (Cant and Sharma, 1999). As in orthodox medicine in the 19th century, the rapidity and extent of professionalisation may be influenced by social exclusion agendas. To judge by the greater comparative marginality among CAM therapies in the UK of traditional Chinese medicine and ayurvedic medicine, which are popular with Asian people, the social exclusion agenda linked to professionalisation may also have ethnic dimensions. The influential House of Lords report on CAM (2000) reinforces this view, in that these therapies are depicted as the least credible CAM practices and are negatively categorised together with iridology and radionics.

4.5 The future: advantages and disadvantages of professionalisation

The House of Lords report on CAM (2000) also gives some insight into the potential future of professionalisation in this field. One of several recommendations that this crucial report makes is that there should be a coherent professional framework for CAM, with specific arrangements for each therapy. It argues that CAM therapies such as acupuncture and herbal medicine are now ready to join the ranks of osteopathy and chiropractic in being granted statutory regulation because of:

- the risks to patients from unqualified practitioners
- the well-organised voluntary regulatory systems that exist in these areas
- the desire of most CAM practitioners in such fields to move to statutory regulation
- the extent of the underpinning research base.

As pointed out in Chapter 3, the report holds that other, less hazardous CAM therapies should be based on the model of voluntary self-regulation, with suitable competency and training guidelines. It also claims that more independent accreditation boards and greater standardisation of courses linked to higher education should be established in this process. It believes that training in subjects on the curriculum of the medical profession should only be incorporated into CAM programmes where its practitioners are operating as mainstream, as opposed to adjunct, therapists. However, it is emphasised that all CAM practitioners should be trained in research methods and given clear instruction on when medical referral is necessary; conversely, those in medical and other orthodox health professions should be familiarised with the use of CAM therapies.

In this respect, the House of Lords Select Committee judged that all NHS provision in CAM should be accessed by referral from orthodox health professionals. It also held that, where there is strong evidence for particular types of CAM, the medical profession should ensure that the public can access them. The report acknowledges that more research may be required into the comparative efficacy, safety and cost-effectiveness of CAM therapies, which should be supported partly by the Department of Health and disseminated to the public as appropriate. The underlying model, though, is one of professional control of CAM in the state sector, which is also supported by the BMA (1993).

In summary, the House of Lords report paints a bright picture of the future for professionalising CAM, even if it believes that a variety of forms are necessary, including the model of medical professional control of CAM therapies within the NHS. As far as groups of non-medical CAM practitioners are concerned, it recommends that the forms of professionalisation range from statutory regulation to voluntary self-regulation, depending on factors such as the evidence for the therapy and the level of danger to the patient. The recent reform of the Health Professions Council, with the removal of the restriction on the number of associated professions, now makes it easier to enact legislation for CAM in statutory areas.

The pros and cons of professionalisation for the public

A key issue is whether the professionalisation of CAM is advantageous to the public, given the growing demand for greater access to such therapies. This also relates back to the theories of the professions outlined in Section 4.2 and how the work of functionalist writers depicted professionalisation in a positive light. This was because of the perceived benefits of, among other features, more robust educational provision, enhanced expertise, and peer regulation of ethics in areas of high importance to society. In this respect, greater degrees of professionalisation of CAM on the appropriate terms would certainly make collaboration more attractive to the medical profession and relevant employing organisations – particularly in terms of assuring the quality of supply in the face of potential litigation – and thereby increase its integration in the NHS (Stone and Matthews, 1996). This in turn would further open up the public's access to CAM, given that it is currently primarily concentrated in the private sector (Saks, 2003).

However, while advantages to the public from the professionalisation of CAM can be acknowledged within a neo-Weberian perspective, these are typically seen as coincidental, the main driver being the political resolution of occupational interests in the power struggles over professionalisation. As previously noted, this is apparent in the adversarial history of the relationship between orthodox medicine and CAM practitioners. Similarly, the professional control of CAM by doctors through referral relationships and the biomedical training of CAM practitioners advocated by the House of Lords report (2000) may accord with medical interests but they are not necessarily most desirable for the public. Doctors may, for example, currently have too little knowledge of CAM to perform a gatekeeping role effectively, which could impose unnecessary limits on its use. As discussed in Chapter 2, training CAM therapists in biomedicine may also have a detrimental effect on access to more holistic forms of CAM (see Box 4.6). These are not always compatible with the philosophy of orthodox medicine, which tends to view the patient as a symptom-bearing organism, hierarchically subordinated to the expert practitioner (Saks, 2003).

BOX 4.6   THE MEDICAL PROFESSION AND HOLISTIC FORMS OF CAM

Saks (1997) notes that while orthodox medicine is not without its holistic aspects — as highlighted, for instance, by the present broad definition of public health and the stress on enhanced communication with patients — some forms of CAM are more holistic because they are strongly based on such features as:

- personalised diagnosis and treatment
- a whole person approach linking mind and body
- meeting the psychological, spiritual and emotional needs of the individual
- considering environmental influences on the client
- greater client participation or involvement
- client self-responsibility for health.

Although not all types of CAM are holistic, bringing such practices within the more reductionist biomedical control of doctors may risk prejudicing these elements of CAM.

It is worth stressing that other stakeholders stand to benefit from the professionalisation of CAM in the terms described in the House of Lords report. These include orthodox health professions and especially leading elements of the medical profession. Clearly, more medical professional control over CAM would advance their interests in relation to income, status and power. The great upsurge of public demand for CAM, backed by significant political support, means the outright rejection of CAM by orthodox medicine is no longer an option. However, medical incorporation – whether through sub-delegation to or by health professions or other means – gives doctors the opportunity to limit the activity of CAM practitioners, while expanding the territory that they themselves can colonise (for example, see Saks, 1992 on acupuncture).

Also, do not forget that some groups of CAM practitioners are potentially advantaged by professionalising in terms of their interests, even within the framework of medical control. This is because the effects of professional closure enhance the position of such groups in the marketplace, thereby providing opportunities for increasing their own income, status and power. In addition, the enhanced educational infrastructure associated with this process protects them from being excluded from practice in the wake of the increasing harmonisation of professional regulation across Europe – at a time when, unlike in the UK, most other European countries exclude non-medical CAM therapists from practice (Huggon and Trench, 1992).

The positive advantages of professional legitimation for CAM by association with the public image of the medical profession are no more intriguingly illustrated than by the choice of spirit guides by Harry Edwards, one of the most famous spiritual healers in the UK. He treated many thousands of intractable cases in the mid-20th century by the laying on of hands. Inglis (1980) notes that, despite the unconventional nature of his practice, the spirit guides he selected could not have been more orthodox. They were Louis Pasteur and Joseph Lister – the founding fathers of biomedicine in the 19th century.

Note that not all CAM practitioners see professionalisation as an attractive way forward. Aside from potentially creating barriers to reciprocal collaborative and egalitarian relationships with clients, there is a widespread aversion to following a model of professionalism that may simply lead to more self-interested protectionism – as such practitioners frequently perceive is the case in orthodox medicine. There are also concerns among CAM therapists about practising as professionals within the NHS, as many such practitioners originally entered the field on an apprenticeship model, to work individually in private practice and avoid bureaucratic constraints (Sharma, 1995).

4.6   Conclusion

This chapter moved from broad issues concerning political power and professionalisation to the more specific health professional context in the UK in which power struggles over professionalisation in both orthodox medicine and CAM were analysed. In weighing up the advantages and disadvantages of professionalisation in CAM, a new model of professionalism could evolve that avoids most of the pitfalls of the traditional concept of a profession,

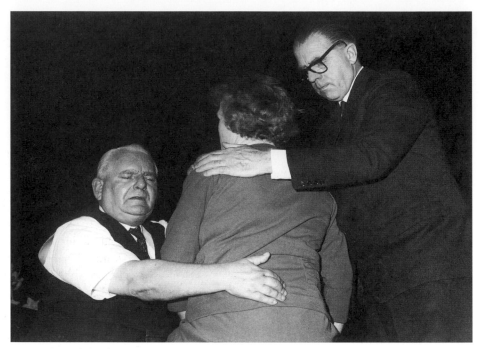

Harry Edwards healing a patient in the 1950s

while drawing on its strongest virtues in terms of public protection. However, what the future holds from a neo-Weberian perspective is most likely to be based on the exercise of political power in the ongoing battles among occupational interests in the wider socioeconomic environment, as several groups of CAM therapists vie with the dominant medical profession and allied health professions in striving to gain an acceptable level of professional standing.

Future developments in the UK in professionalisation in the health field in general and CAM in particular will be of no less interest as they ebb and flow in a field that continues to be heavily shaped by conflict and political power.

KEY POINTS

- The meaning of 'profession' and 'professionalisation' is contested.
- There are several different mainstream theories of the professions, ranging from the earlier positive to more recent critical perspectives.
- The politicised neo-Weberian approach is used to discuss the development of the medical profession, the allied professions and CAM in the UK. This approach focuses on professions as groups that seek to promote and serve their own interests.
- Historically, the professionalisation of medicine and other orthodox health professions has had a detrimental impact on CAM.
- The initial blockades to the professionalisation of CAM are being overcome by the upsurge of popular and political support for CAM.
- Several CAM therapies are at various stages in the process of professionalisation and some involve the medical incorporation of CAM.
- The future of CAM professionalisation in the UK is now under consideration, especially since the House of Lords report.
- There are advantages and disadvantages to different stakeholder groups of professionalising CAM.

References

Allsop, J. (1995) 'Shifting spheres of opportunity: the professional powers of general practitioners within the British National Health Service', in Johnson, T., Larkin, G. and Saks, M. (eds) *Health Professions and the State in Europe*, London, Routledge.

Allsop, J. (2002) 'Regulation and the medical profession', in Allsop, J. and Saks, M. (eds) *Regulating the Health Professions*, London, Sage.

Allsop, J. and Saks, M. (2002) 'Introduction: the regulation of health professions', in Allsop, J. and Saks, M. (eds) *Regulating the Health Professions*, London, Sage.

Barber, B. (1963) 'Some problems in the sociology of professions', *Daedalus*, Vol. 92, pp. 669–88.

Becker, H. (1962) 'The nature of a profession', in National Society for the Study of Education (ed.) *Education for the Professions*, Chicago, MI, University of Chicago.

Berlant, J. L. (1975) *Profession and Monopoly: A Study of Medicine in the United States and Great Britain*, Berkeley, CA, University of California Press.

British Medical Association (1993) *Complementary Medicine: New Approaches to Good Practice*, London, BMA.

Cant, S. and Sharma, U. (1995) *Professionalization in Complementary Medicine*, Report on a research project funded by the Economic and Social Research Council, London.

Cant, S. and Sharma, U. (1996) 'Demarcation and transformation within homoeopathic knowledge: a strategy of professionalization', *Social Science and Medicine*, Vol. 42, pp. 579–88.

Cant, S. and Sharma, U. (1999) *A New Medical Pluralism? Alternative Medicine, Doctors, Patients and the State*, London, UCL Press.

Davies, C. (2002) 'Registering a difference: changes in the regulation of nursing', in Allsop, J. and Saks, M. (eds) *Regulating the Health Professions*, London, Sage.

Elston, M. (1991) 'The politics of professional power: medicine in a changing health service', in Gabe, J., Calnan, M. and Bury, M. (eds) *The Sociology of the Health Service*, London, Routledge.

Esland, G. (1980) 'Diagnosis and therapy', in Esland, G. and Salaman, G. (eds) *The Politics of Work and Occupations*, pp. 251–78, Milton Keynes, Open University Press.

Etzioni, A. (ed.) (1969) *The Semi-Professions and Their Organization*, New York, Free Press.

Foucault, M. (1980) *Power/Knowledge*, Brighton, Harvester Press.

Freidson, E. (1970) *Profession of Medicine*, New York, Dodd, Mead & Co.

Freidson, E. (1983) 'The theory of professions – state of the art', in Dingwall, R. and Lewis, P. (eds) *The Sociology of Professions*, London, Macmillan.

Fulder, S. (1996) *The Handbook of Alternative and Complementary Medicine* (3rd edn), Oxford, Oxford University Press.

Goode, W. (1960) 'Encroachment, charlatanism and the emerging profession: psychology, sociology and medicine', *American Sociological Review*, Vol. 25, pp. 902–14.

House of Lords (2000) Select Committee on Science and Technology's Sixth Report, *Complementary and Alternative Medicine*, London, The Stationery Office.

Huggon, T. and Trench, A. (1992) 'Brussels post-1992: protector or persecutor?', in Saks, M. (ed.) *Alternative Medicine in Britain*, Oxford, Clarendon Press.

Hughes, E. (1963) 'Professions', *Daedalus*, Vol. 92, pp. 655–68.

Inglis, B. (1980) *Natural Medicine*, London, Fontana.

Johnson, T. (1972) *Professions and Power*, London, Macmillan.

Jones, L. J. (1994) *The Social Context of Health and Health Work*, Basingstoke, Macmillan.

Larkin, G. (1983) *Occupational Monopoly and Modern Medicine*, London, Tavistock.

Larkin, G. (1992) 'Orthodox and osteopathic medicine in the inter-war years', in Saks, M. (ed.) *Alternative Medicine in Britain*, Oxford, Clarendon Press.

Larkin, G. (1995) 'State control and the health professions in the United Kingdom: historical perspectives', in Johnson, T., Larkin, G. and Saks, M. (eds) *Health Professions and the State in Europe*, London, Routledge.

Larkin, G. (2002) 'The regulation of the professions allied to medicine', in Allsop, J. and Saks, M. (eds) *Regulating the Health Professions*, London, Sage.

Millerson, G. (1964) *The Qualifying Associations*, London, Routledge & Kegan Paul.

Navarro, V. (1986) *Crisis, Health and Medicine: A Social Critique*, London, Tavistock.

Nettleton, S. (1992) *Power, Pain and Dentistry*, Buckingham, Open University Press.

Parkin, F. (1979) *Marxism and Class Theory: A Bourgeois Critique*, London, Tavistock.

Parry, N. and Parry, J. (1977) 'Social closure and collective social mobility', in Scase, R. (ed.) *Industrial Society: Class, Cleavage and Control*, London, Allen & Unwin.

Parsons, T. (1951) *The Social System*, New York, Free Press.

Poulantzas, N. (1975) *Classes in Contemporary Capitalism*, London, New Left Books.

Roth, J. (1974) 'Professionalism: the sociologist's decoy', *Sociology of Work and Occupations*, Vol. 1, pp. 6–23.

Saks, M. (1992) 'The paradox of incorporation: acupuncture and the medical profession in modern Britain', in Saks, M. (ed.) *Alternative Medicine in Britain*, Oxford, Clarendon Press.

Saks, M. (1995) *Professions and the Public Interest: Professional Power, Altruism and Alternative Medicine*, London, Routledge.

Saks, M. (1996) 'From quackery to complementary medicine: the shifting boundaries between orthodox and unorthodox medical knowledge', in Cant, S. and Sharma, U. (eds) *Complementary and Alternative Medicines: Knowledge in Practice*, London, Free Association Books.

Saks, M. (1997) 'Alternative therapies: are they holistic?', *Complementary Therapies in Nursing and Midwifery*, Vol. 3, pp. 4–8.

Saks, M. (1999) 'The wheel turns? Professionalisation and alternative medicine in Britain', *Journal of Interprofessional Care*, Vol. 13, pp. 129–38.

Saks, M. (2000) 'Medicine and the counter culture', in Cooter, R. and Pickstone, J. (eds) *Medicine in the Twentieth Century*, Amsterdam, Harwood Academic Publishers.

Saks, M. (2001) 'Alternative medicine and the health care division of labour: present trends and future prospects', *Current Sociology*, Vol. 49, pp. 119–34.

Saks, M. (2002) 'Professionalisation, regulation and alternative medicine', in Allsop, J. and Saks, M. (eds) *Regulating the Health Professions*, London, Sage.

Saks, M. (2003) *Orthodox and Alternative Medicine: Politics, Professionalization and Health Care*, London, Sage.

Sharma, U. (1995) *Complementary Medicine Today: Practitioners and Patients* (revised edition), London, Routledge.

Stacey, M. (1988) *The Sociology of Health and Healing*, London, Unwin Hyman.

Stacey, M. (1992) *Regulating British Medicine: The General Medical Council*, Chichester, John Wiley & Sons.

Stone, J. and Matthews, J. (1996) *Complementary Medicine and the Law*, Oxford, Oxford University Press.

Turner, B. (1995) *Medical Power and Social Knowledge* (2nd edition), London, Sage.

Wallis, R. and Morley, P. (1976) 'Introduction', in Wallis, R. and Morley, P. (eds) *Marginal Medicine*, London, Peter Owen.

Weber, M. (1968) *Economy and Society* (first published 1922), New York, Bedminster Press.

Witz, A. (1992) *Professions and Patriarchy*, London, Routledge.

Chapter 5 Homeopathy: principles, practice and controversies

Phil Nicholls, Geraldine Lee-Treweek and Tom Heller

Contents

AIMS

- To describe the history and practice of homeopathy.
- To use the study of homeopathy to illustrate themes relating more generally to CAM philosophy and practice.

5.1 Introduction

In this chapter homeopathy, a popular and well-known form of complementary medicine in the UK, is used to explore the issues raised in Chapters 1 to 4. Homeopathy is an interesting example of how the philosophy and practice of complementary and alternative medicine (CAM) can appear to contradict orthodox scientific principles and yet still remain popular with both the general public and the increasing numbers of orthodox practitioners who are integrating CAM into their practice. In many high street pharmacies and health food shops, homeopathic remedies can be bought over the counter or there is a ready availability of homeopathic practitioners to consult in person. Homeopathy has been integrated into the National Health Service (NHS) in the form of the Royal Homoeopathic Hospitals and through its use by general practitioners, nurses and others in a variety of NHS settings. Indeed, homeopathy is classified as one of the 'Big Five' modalities that are considered to be complementary to and congruent with contemporary orthodox health provision (House of Lords, 2000). Yet, at the same time, homeopathic theories remain consistently challenging to orthodox concepts of health and currently accepted processes of disease, illness and treatment.

This chapter begins by discussing the central tenets of this popular CAM modality. The founder of homeopathy, Dr Samuel Hahnemann, developed a group of principles that are unique to homeopathic medicine. These include the notion that 'like treats like', the use of symptom pictures and pathways, and the dilution and dynamisation of remedies.

The chapter goes on to trace the history of the shifting boundaries between homeopathy and orthodox medicine from its beginning to the present day. It raises some interesting questions about the education and training of CAM practitioners.

The chapter ends with a discussion of the way in which homeopathy, whose basic principles do not fit with orthodox science, has been the focus of much scepticism. The question of whether homeopathy works is examined and the processes by which claims of fraud have been made are explored.

5.2   Hahnemann's basic principles in practice

Homeopathy is a highly popular form of CAM in the UK. The World Health Organization estimates that homeopathy is the second most popular CAM therapy in the world, practised in about 67 countries, with approximately 300 million users (WHO, 2004).

In the UK, homeopathic remedies can be bought over the counter at major pharmacies, and numerous books and self-help guides can be used to deduce the remedy needed. Users may also choose to consult a homeopathic practitioner for a detailed consultation and the prescription of homeopathic remedies. However, at the same time as enjoying this popularity, homeopathy continues to challenge two fundamental principles of orthodox medicine. Whereas orthodox medicine attempts to oppose the symptoms of disease, homeopathy encourages them; and whereas orthodox medicine treats patients with measurable, material quantities of potent drugs, homeopathy uses medicines at such high levels of dilution that usually no trace of the 'active' ingredient is detectable.

The development and principles of homeopathy

The German physician Samuel Hahnemann (1755–1843) first developed homeopathy as a discrete system of medicine from the 1790s onwards. The word 'homoeopathy' (now more usually spelt 'homeopathy') is derived from the Greek words for 'like' (*homoios*) and 'suffering' (*pathos*). Homeopathy involves a gentle form of treatment that some critics argue is so gentle it cannot possibly work. It is interesting to consider the setting in which Hahnemann developed homeopathy. Many of the treatments of the day, used

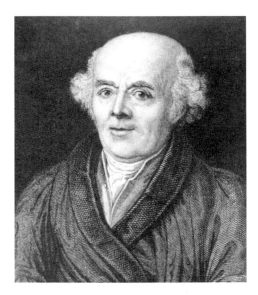

Samuel Hahnemann, the founder of homeopathy

on sick people by doctors or prescribed by pharmacists, had extreme effects on the body. Doctors and pharmacists were used to prescribing and compounding powerful doses of purgative drugs (such as arsenic and mercury), and to bleeding and blistering their patients. These extreme and painful treatments produced demonstrable effects; the users could see that something was happening to their body. In essence, such practitioners could demonstrate their expertise through the effects of their treatments and people felt they were getting their money's worth. However, the effects of such treatments on overall health could be injurious to the person being treated. At the same time, there was a considerable struggle for power between different types of practitioner in the medical marketplace. From the point when Hahnemann first published *The Organon of Rational Healing* – his definitive statement of homeopathic theory and practice – in 1810, he became embroiled in controversy over his new theories and gentle treatments. Other practitioners opposed Hahnemann and ridiculed homeopathy at every opportunity.

For orthodox doctors, there was more at stake than mere theoretical difference. Homeopathy rapidly gained in popularity among patients and, even more crucially, became fashionable among the social elites of the UK, continental Europe and the USA. Homeopathy had to be ridiculed not merely because it seemed absurd to materialist thinking, but also because it threatened the incomes of orthodox medical practitioners whose livelihoods depended on maintaining the loyalty of paying customers. The competition from homeopathic doctors was particularly unwelcome in a profession that was usually overcrowded, and where initiatives were begun, from the mid-19th century onwards, to improve the status, income, education and professional standing of medical practitioners as a whole.

How did Hahnemann come to develop his unique therapeutic system? The answer seems to lie in his experience as a medical practitioner. After graduating in 1779, Hahnemann became progressively concerned about the disabling and detrimental effects on patients of powerful drugs (such as mercury) and treatments that weakened the patient (such as phlebotomy or bleeding). His anxiety was sufficient to persuade him, in about 1782, to stop practising medicine and to earn his living instead as a translator, writer and chemical researcher. During this period of his life he was commissioned, in 1790, to translate into German the work of the famous Scottish physician William Cullen. In Cullen's *Treatise of the Materia Medica* (1789), Hahnemann came across the author's explanation for the efficacy of the popular drug known as 'Peruvian bark' or 'China' from the tree *Cinchona officinalis* (the bark contains the anti-malarial drug quinine). Cullen attributed the drug's efficacy in cases of fever to its astringent and bitter qualities which, he argued, helped to restore normal 'tone' to a hot and feverish body. Hahnemann disagreed with Cullen's explanation – on the quite reasonable grounds that a remedy could be made that was far more 'bitter' and 'astringent' than 'the bark', and yet it would have no fever-calming properties at all.

Let likes be treated by likes: treatment by similarity

To understand the therapeutic properties of *Cinchona*, Hahnemann then experimented by taking four drams of the medicine twice daily for several days. He carefully noted the symptoms he experienced. His records convinced him that the symptoms the drug had produced actually **matched** the symptoms of the disease that the drug normally helped to cure. Thus the homeopathic principle of *similia similibus curentur* – let likes be treated by likes – was born.

ACTIVITY   MATCHING SIMILARS

Allow 10 minutes

To understand this first principle of homeopathy further, consider the three symptoms listed below. What substance in your opinion might produce a similar effect or the actual symptom? For example, peeling onions could produce watery eyes.

(a)   Sore throat

(b)   Headache

(c)   Heartburn

Comment

You may have thought of a whole range of suggestions for how these symptoms could be produced. A sore throat could result from eating hot, spicy food; a headache from having too much to drink; and heartburn again from eating spicy foods but also rich or highly acidic foods. Homeopathic remedies harness the power of similars to make the body combat illness for itself. You may think this is similar to vaccination and, indeed, vaccination uses a similar idea. However, as shown later in this section, homeopaths use similar substances at far lower potencies than any inoculation and their ideas about what happens to the body are also different.

Hahnemann spent the years that followed his experiment elaborating and refining the homeopathic system. His experience with *Cinchona* persuaded him that the key to identifying the therapeutic domain of drugs was to 'prove' potential remedies on healthy people. Hahnemann used himself, his friends and family to 'prove' his new remedies. Detailed records were made of the physical and mental symptoms experienced by 'provers' after the drug was administered, and a 'picture' of the drug was established from the resulting data. The principle of treatment by similarity then indicated the cases in which the drug should be used. When a detailed picture of the signs and symptoms of a sick patient matched those produced by a drug on healthy people, the correct remedy for the patient had been established. Ill people would be treated with a drug that could give them the same symptoms if they were well. Hahnemann developed his idea that it was clearly of utmost importance to collect detailed information about the sick person to get the remedy absolutely right. By the time he died, in 1843, he had supervised the proving of some 99 medicines in this way. Now thousands of remedies have been 'proved' and are used for homeopathic treatment.

> For example, a homeopath would treat a patient with a cold whose primary symptoms are lacrimation, stinging and irritation of the eyes, and thin, clear nasal discharge with a potency prepared from onion extracts (*Allium cepa*) because these symptoms mimic those produced by onions. However, another patient with a cold might have thick, yellow nasal discharge, have lost all thirst, and want cool, fresh air. That person would be treated with a potency of the purple cone flower (*Pulsatilla*) because these symptoms are more characteristic of those produced by this plant.
>
> (Jonas et al., 2003, p. 393)

Symptom pictures and pathways

Hahnemann explained why the treatment of 'likes by likes' appeared to work by resorting to the idea of the healing power of Nature or, as he called it, 'the vital force'. In essence, he argued that the human organism has a natural impulse to heal itself, and that the signs and symptoms of illness in individual patients represent the 'picture' or 'pathway' chosen by the body in its struggle to regain health. The physician's role, therefore, must be to support the body's own recuperative strategy by administering medicines which gently stimulate the healing process. This is achieved using the similar remedy. One of the most important consequences of this notion of individual pictures or pathways is that different people fight disease in individual and different ways. Therefore, the homeopath should support the body in fighting disease in the way it chooses and not prescribe a fixed medicine for each disease (Castro, 1990).

Hahnemann's ideas emphasise the need for a holistic approach that may mean people with the same disease are prescribed very different medicines. As each person fights disease differently, it is imperative to find the right remedy. Such an approach emphasises the meticulous and rigorous collection of information from the ill person because they will be given one remedy at a time and this remedy should match all their physical and mental symptoms. Such a match will also include individual likes and dislikes, fears and worries and even emotions. In this way the remedy is suitably matched to **the individual** and not to a particular disease. In homeopathic thinking it is more than 'personality' or 'characteristic ways of fighting disease' that distinguish each individual and their response to disease. This concept constitutes a major difference from biomedicine, although it could be argued that modern knowledge of the ways in which genetic inheritance predisposes people to certain kinds of disease constitutes a potential area of 'convergence'.

Another idea that is important to the practice of homeopathy is that illness or disease often has layers. This means that whereas a person with one ailment may consult a homeopath, the alleviation of this problem could lead to another ailment (which has been dormant for years) surfacing after the first one disappears. This raises the issue of how the success of treatment can be judged against that which orthodox health care practitioners might use. For example, if a person with chronic headaches goes to a homeopath they may be given a particular remedy that suits their personality and individual symptom picture. However, they may find that the headaches go but bloating and constipation develop instead. The homeopath may view this as another layer of the first illness rather than seeing the treatment as a failure or the new symptoms as a new illness. This process of revealing symptoms may go on for a long time and some homeopaths would argue that, in part, these layers represent the suppression of illness through orthodox treatments over the course of the individual's life. Many non-medically qualified (NMQ) homeopaths believe that biomedical treatment can be actively harmful for patients, even if in the short term the presenting symptoms disappear, because it suppresses symptoms.

Dilution and 'dynamisation' of remedies

Hahnemann took his theories further. He added the principle of **potentisation** or **dynamisation** of remedies to the principle of treatment by a similar remedy. Hahnemann argued that to stimulate the non-material vital force of the body, remedies have to be prepared in a way that releases their own healing energy. This process involves taking one part of the drug itself, adding it to 99 parts of distilled water, vigorously shaking (or 'succussing') the two together, and then repeating the sequence by taking one part of the first dilution and adding that again to 99 parts of distilled water (see Box 5.1).

BOX 5.1   MAKING SENSE OF HOMEOPATHIC DOSAGES

The dosage of homeopathic remedies is often written on the packaging. Typically these are 6C or 30C, although homeopathic practitioners often prescribe dosages up to 200C. A 6C preparation is a 1 to 10 dilution repeated six times. This leaves the active ingredient at 1 part per million. In homeopathic philosophy, the less active the ingredient, the stronger the homeopathic drug. So 200C is seen homeopathically as more potent in its action than 6C, despite the fact that the former potency is more dilute. However, it is not just the dilution that is important. The key to the strength lies in the succussions between the dilutions that homeopaths believe activate the healing properties of the liquid. They would argue that this liquid contains the imprint or essence of the substance, even if there appears to be no ingredients left in relation to orthodox scientific methods and measurement. Once the liquid is at the right potency, it is dripped on to sugar pills. These remedies tend to be much cheaper than many orthodox drugs and, it is claimed, people cannot overdose on them.

Once this process has been repeated 13 times, the resulting solution almost certainly does not contain any detectable trace of the original active ingredient. However, homeopaths were to go   and continue to go – far beyond 13 dilutions. Indeed, homeopathic preparations are graded according to the number of succussions and homeopaths believe the more dilutions there are, the more potent is the remedy. This means in practice that a remedy is considered to be stronger the weaker it is, which may mean diluting 100 times beyond there being any detectable substance left in the distilled water! This water is then dripped on to sugar tablets, which are given to the person attending for treatment. As homeopaths believe very little remedy is needed, they often advise taking the medication once a day, once a week or even once a month. For example, in the case of a chest infection getting worse, an orthodox doctor is unlikely to prescribe fewer antibiotics but rather more, or a stronger dose, or a different type of antibiotic. However, in homeopathic practice, slightly worsening symptoms are often hailed as a good sign: it indicates that the remedy is working, the body is responding and healing is beginning.

Homeopathy: old criticisms and new remedies

Homeopathy continues to court controversy for similar reasons to those in Hahnemann's time. Its opponents claim that homeopathy simply cannot work. As a set of ideas about the world and how it works, homeopathy

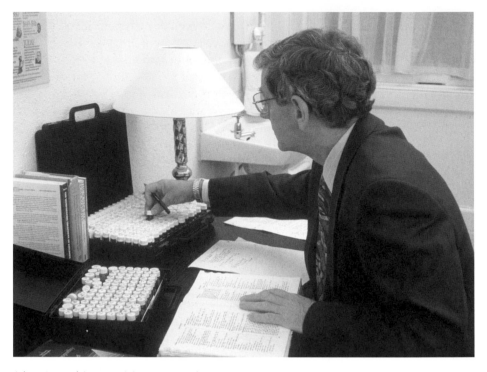

A homeopathic practitioner at work

challenges basic scientific principles. For instance, according to orthodox science, its remedies are inert because, after the multiple dilutions, modern chemistry cannot detect any of the original substance or medicine left. For orthodox medicine, which relies on the idea of increasing doses of medicines to treat more severe cases of disease, the idea of using less remedy, and minuscule amounts at that, does not make sense. For many critics the answer to why people continue to use homeopathy and seem to get well rests on the nature of the homeopathic consultation, the relationship between the practitioner and user of homeopathy, or the user's belief in the treatment. In short, it is argued, reassurance from the practitioner and confidence in a good outcome by the user may lead to the user feeling and getting better – the result of the placebo effect, which is discussed in Chapter 6.

The same claim about a placebo effect can be made of people who buy over-the-counter (OTC) homeopathic remedies because their expectations may positively affect the outcome. Another point about OTC treatment is that people who buy such remedies are unlikely to be very ill. Indeed, many such remedies are designed to treat transient symptoms that will probably get better by themselves over time, for example heartburn, aches and pains and bruising. It is difficult for the person buying the treatment to know whether the homeopathic preparation made them better or whether they would have recovered in time anyway.

Homeopaths have tried to use evidence derived from controlled clinical trials of their remedies to resist the claim that any demonstrated effect is merely placebo. Such studies have been accumulating since the 1980s. There are now some 93 such trials in the published medical literature (Mathie, 2003), and around 50 of them claim to demonstrate a positive treatment effect. Where such an effect is demonstrated, and where a trial is properly designed and controlled, the results seem to challenge established principles of physics and chemistry, and present the scientific community with a dilemma. If homeopathic theory is correct, some of the basic principles of orthodox medicine may therefore be wrong. One possible response in this situation is to claim that fraud or trickery must have been used to produce the outcomes. These claims are examined in Section 5.4. One factor that magnifies the potential placebo effect of homeopathic remedies is the extensive and intensive nature of the usual consultation process with a homeopathic practitioner. Such therapists are either medically qualified doctors, with a postgraduate qualification from the Faculty of Homoeopathy, or 'professional' homeopaths who, although lacking medical certification, have been trained at a homeopathic college. The Society of Homeopaths prefers the term 'professional' homeopath for NMQ practitioners to 'lay'. But, whether medically qualified or 'professional', the practitioner will spend considerable time establishing a detailed, precise and individual symptom picture of the presenting person. This is critical because the very idiosyncrasy of a particular person's symptom complex is the key to finding the correct remedy:

> A homeopathic consultation is time consuming; the practitioner will explore personal and family history, physical symptoms, social circumstances, and emotional issues with her patient ... always looking for the unusual symptoms or characteristics which will point to the correct remedy. Thus, she is, by definition, interested in the patient as an individual. Thus, the sort of in-depth, respectful attention which feminist critics have wanted from their health care providers is a necessary part of homeopathic practice.
>
> (Scott, 1998, p. 205)

This in-depth assessment of the patient is one of the key differences between choosing to self-medicate with OTC homeopathic remedies (which are now so readily available from high street chemists) or using remedies prescribed by a homeopath. In the latter case, the remedy is, as it were, 'tailor-made' to match the person's unique symptom picture. Many OTC homeopathic remedies, however, tend to give indications for use which **do** focus on classes of disease. This is perhaps understandable for commercial retailers but it is not really 'homeopathy' since homeopaths do not prescribe on the basis of disease categories but, rather, on the individual symptom picture presented by a unique person.

The uniqueness of people's symptom pictures has led homeopaths to continue to search for, prove and then add new remedies to their pharmacopoeia (an encyclopaedia of medicines). New remedies can be made from animal, mineral or vegetable materials. However, Hahnemann's basic principles remain the same and the remedies are developed through dilutions in the same way. Among the latest remedies to be introduced by homeopaths are bird remedies (Hardy, 2003). These are prepared from the feathers, claws or blood of different birds. The symbolism in the provings is significant: feelings of lightness, freedom, responsibility, danger, intuition and a desire for travel have been frequently reported in healthy individuals who took bird remedies.

A specific example of one of these new remedies gives a sense of the evocative nuances of homeopathic drug pictures, and perhaps also of the appeal and fascination of homeopathy to its practitioners. This remedy is made from the homeopathically processed essence of peregrine falcon feathers:

> The central theme in this remedy is a deep sense of isolation. There is a very strong feeling of being excluded. The patient feels neglected and repudiated by friends, family and society as a whole. ... There is a very negative self-image with feelings of disgust at oneself and at one's body, a feeling of ugliness ... of shame, humiliation and resentment. ... These feelings can lead to a deep sense of hopelessness and apathy. The patient may become discontented, discouraged, indifferent and lazy.
>
> (Hardy, 2003, p. 8)

Someone with this symptom picture would be treated with the remedy (using the rule that 'like cures like'). Note that this remedy is not for a disease or a specific illness: it is solely for treating a range of diverse symptoms. In this case, the remedy is heavily related to feelings, emotions, doubts and personality and is another example of how the homeopathic practitioner is involved with painstakingly collecting information from the person and then matching symptoms to seek the correct homeopathic remedy. Some homeopathic practitioners argue against the use of bird remedies, claiming that it is not homeopathy. They suggest that the development of a new homeopathic remedy must involve the procedure Samuel Hahnemann used more than 200 years ago: that is, see whether an undiluted substance causes the same symptoms in many people with good health. For example, to evaluate the symptoms caused by a mosquito, use the poison of the insect not the wings to claim the remedy could be effective against insect bites rather than a fear of flying.

ACTIVITY   REASONS FOR THE POPULARITY OF HOMEOPATHY

Allow 20 minutes

How many reasons can you think of for the current popularity of homeopathy in the UK? You need to think about what homeopathy offers its users in comparison with other forms of medicine.

Comment

Your reasons may have included some of the following.

- The low doses appeal to people who dislike taking conventional drugs. Homeopathy is alleged to be a safe form of treatment for everyone because of the low doses and dilution.

- The remedies involved are relatively cheap and may not have to be taken very often.

- The centrally important role of the therapeutic relationship may explain homeopathy's popularity because people are given personal attention and time to discuss their problems.

- Access to homeopathy is easy. Homeopathic preparations are available in most high street pharmacies as well as practitioners who offer treatment throughout the UK.

- There are many resources for people who want to treat themselves homeopathically, from internet sites that help find the correct remedy to home guides that are available in most health food stores and general bookshops.

- As with many other modalities, homeopathy frees users from the constraint of details going on their medical records. Some of the problems treated by homeopaths include emotional or psychological distress and, for reasons of privacy, users may be particularly attracted by not having to use orthodox care.

5.3   Diverse histories and challenged boundaries

Using remedies derived from bits of birds may appear to put homeopathy firmly in the camp of alternative or 'fringe' medicine. However, it is difficult to label something as marginal when it is so popular. Also, such labels are often given to various CAM modalities by people who want to play down the importance of a competitor. In response, some homeopaths have attempted to rescue their credibility by using exactly the same scientific procedures in the form of a clinical trial to show that their remedies do have demonstrable therapeutic activity (Mathie, 2003).

However, this apparently simple solution to the problem of what counts as 'alternative' medicine ignores the fact that the practice of science is a social process. Indeed, this chapter will argue that the way in which boundaries between orthodox medicine and CAM are drawn is as much the product of social, personal and political struggles as it is the outcome of neutral scientific procedures. To clarify this, it is useful to take a historical perspective in order to show how such boundaries were drawn in 18th and 19th-century Britain.

Any notion of a distinct boundary between regular and 'quack' or fringe medicine in the 18th century is misconceived. As Porter (1999) argues, the 18th-century medical marketplace was competitive and commercialised, and in the doctor–patient relationship the client or patron tended to be the dominant partner. The structure of patron or client relationships meant that practitioners sought to diversify therapeutic methods and theories and to advertise their individuality. There was little material basis for any sense of strong professional solidarity. The educated gentleman – the typical patient of the physicians of the day – could be expected to know as much about medicine as the doctor, could negotiate treatment, and wielded considerable economic and social power over him.

However, in the 19th century, conditions emerged which changed physician–client relationships. Industrialisation, population growth and urbanisation created new medical markets, especially among the new middle classes, and underpinned the development and expansion of voluntary hospitals. These were the new sites where medical power began to develop. Crucially, voluntary hospitals were charitable institutions designed for the relief of poor, working-class patients who had little ability to defend themselves against medical dominance. It was almost the first time that physicians and surgeons could observe patients and make authoritative decisions about patient management as well as gain access to the results of post mortems, which provided the critical opportunity to match visible signs and symptoms with internal pathology. The real issue for medicine at this time was who had the right to practise, and who should control what was practised, rather than a disinterested attempt to evaluate the range of therapeutic instruments or approaches in the interests of patient welfare. After all, in the second half of the 19th century the orthodox profession gradually abandoned heroic therapy. This did not occur because of any objective or controlled investigations showing that it harmed rather than helped. In fact, rival therapies, such as homeopathy, were shunned, despite no systematic evaluations being made of them. So the boundary between 'regular' and 'irregular' practice in medicine is often the outcome of political struggles between different kinds of practitioner, motivated by professional, economic or other factors, rather than a product of a dispassionate appeal to the jury of neutral science.

The first references to the use of homeopathy in the UK appeared in the 1830s. Its first significant practitioner was Hervey Quin (1799–1879), a London-based, fashionable, gentleman doctor with strong connections to the aristocracy. With Quin as an early champion, homeopathy rapidly assumed a high public profile. It soon became fashionable among the clergy and other socially elite groups of the time. From the 1840s onwards, many lay practitioners, as well as qualified doctors, began adopting homeopathy in the UK, mainland Europe and the USA. In an overcrowded profession the financial incentives to adopt homeopathy were considerable.

At first, orthodox medical practitioners treated homeopathy as something of a joke or with disdain. However, the rate of increase in numbers of homeopathic practitioners soon reached a point where it seemed that, within a few years, the profession would be overrun with Hahnemann's followers. Once this future was perceived as real, direct action was taken to eliminate the threat. The result was a political struggle between rival groups of practitioners, motivated by economic and occupational interests rather than scientific 'truth'.

Meanwhile, at the Edinburgh Royal Infirmary, William Henderson, an early pioneer of homeopathy in the UK along with Quin, reported improved recovery rates in his wards through using homeopathic methods. Henderson was probably correct about these benefits to patients, but not necessarily in attributing them to the use of homeopathy: rather it was the absence of the usual hospital rituals of bleeding and purging. The point is, at the time most practitioners were not concerned with these issues. Orthodox medical practitioners were much more interested in the facts that homeopaths were threatening medical incomes and, through the defence of an apparently illogical and indefensible system, undermining professional credibility. In short, a struggle ensued over who had the legitimate right to determine the medical division of labour and to control medical work and education. The orthodox profession's answer was that custom was certainly not to be ceded to the homeopaths and, in pursuit of this political objective, a strategy of ostracism and exclusion was launched. Hospital appointments were withheld from candidates who had practised or supported homeopathy; hospital-based practitioners who were sympathetic to homeopathy found their posts withdrawn; and students who had expressed an interest in homeopathy were prevented from completing their medical training. In addition, some homeopaths were indicted for manslaughter when their patients died, while orthodox doctors refused to consult with homeopaths and evicted them from local branches of the British Medical Association (BMA).

These struggles continued until about the 1880s, by which time they began to lose their force. By then orthodox practitioners had begun to adopt a much less aggressive therapeutic outlook, and so looked more like homeopaths, while homeopaths who were anxious to keep pace with developments in anaesthetics, hygiene and bacteriology began to look more like orthodox practitioners. In short, the reasons for continued hostility had all but disappeared and, towards the end of the 19th century, the ban on BMA membership was lifted, providing any remaining adherents did not publicly proclaim themselves as 'homeopaths'. Co-option had eventually proved to be a better tactic of professional regulation than ostracism. Although medical homeopathy survived as a postgraduate speciality in British medicine, its adherents were too few in number or weak in political voice to present a serious threat. For most of the 20th century, their colleagues in orthodox health care generally regarded medically qualified homeopaths as on the eccentric fringe, still liked by the Royal Family but, for all practical purposes, could be ignored.

Training and change

The 1960s provided the perfect conditions for a return of popular interest in and support for alternative medicine, especially homeopathy. Critics of orthodox medicine began to point to the damaging effects of drug therapy and impersonal treatment. This began the long process through which the status of the traditional 'expert' in modern society was progressively undermined. In addition, the profile of disease had begun to change from acute infections to chronic, lifestyle or degenerative disease requiring more long-term management. CAM modalities such as homeopathy, with their focus on gentle treatments and therapeutic relationships that are often long and involved, have much to offer contemporary health care consumers.

Before the 1960s the fate of homeopathy hung in the balance. Although it had been a popular therapy during the 19th century, at the turn of the century medically trained homeopaths were in decline. Their organisation – The British Homoeopathic Society – had hardly enough members to keep the modality going. This led key medical homeopaths to decide to train lay people so that the modality would not die out. By the 1920s and 1930s there was a growing lay interest but not enough to create a major threat to orthodox care. By the 1970s interest had grown again and, in 1978, a group of lay practitioners established their own Society of Homoeopaths, a register, a college (The London College of Homoeopathy), a journal (*The Homoeopath*) and a code of ethics. At this point the lay and the medical systems of homeopathy were running concurrently. Medically trained homeopaths developed their own body – The Faculty of Homoeopaths – which was designed solely for practitioners with orthodox medical qualifications. Since then the relationship between the two bodies has been based on division and failure to agree on what kind of training a homeopath needs to be an effective and safe practitioner.

ACTIVITY   THE FACULTY OF HOMOEOPATHS AND THE SOCIETY OF HOMOEOPATHS: WORKING TOGETHER?

Allow 30 minutes

Read the excerpt in Box 5.2 from the House of Lords report (2000) and then answer the following questions.

1   What are the main points of the Faculty's arguments against a core curriculum or joint teaching with the Society?
2   What are the key points of the Society's arguments for such joint teaching?

BOX 5.2 A CORE CURRICULUM FOR HOMEOPATHY?

6.91 The Faculty told us that there is very little co-operation between themselves and the Society of Homeopaths over a core curriculum for training homeopaths. Although the Faculty worked on the development of National Occupational Standards in homeopathy they do not train according to the National Occupational Standards. This is because the Faculty believe the training needs of medically qualified homeopathy students are very different from the training needs of those not medically qualified. There are several reasons for this. The Faculty told us: 'In a sense we are not training the same people so a core curriculum for someone starting from scratch to become a homeopath is a completely different training pathway from the core curriculum for a doctor that has done undergraduate training and then postgraduate training'. The Faculty's training therefore assumes that people who come to them for training 'know what the basic foundation of medical science is and know the structure and function of the body and the mechanisms of disease'. The Faculty also believe that medically qualified homeopaths 'do not do the same jobs as people who have not had a medical training. The kind of people who come to a homeopathic hospital will probably of necessity be different from those seeking help in a place where there is no local homeopathic medical provision'. Therefore it would make sense for them to have a slightly different training.

6.92 The Society of Homeopaths agree that '... medical practitioners who have done full medical training do not need to study anatomy, physiology and pathology again'. However they assert that '... to achieve full homeopathic competence — and we are talking here of a philosophical shift of perspective on human health and illness — there is a large block of learning and knowledge to be done which is quite different from conventional medical training and, therefore, we would maintain that to be fully competent homeopathically requires full education and training in the same homeopathic knowledge and understanding that the non-medically qualified homeopaths have'. We are not convinced that this body of knowledge is derived from a firm evidence base.

6.93 The Faculty and the Society agree that previous medical training negates the need for doctors to complete some parts of the course that would be required of non-medical students. It also seems logical that medically qualified individuals may benefit from teaching specifically on how to integrate their two areas of knowledge, conventional and homeopathic. They also agree on the need for an in-depth understanding of the philosophy and practice of homeopathy itself. However, despite what seems to be considerable common ground, the two bodies have had very little communication over what a curriculum needs to include to provide students with no previous knowledge of homeopathy with an in-depth understanding of the practice and philosophy of homeopathy.

(Source: House of Lords, 2000, Chapter 6)

Comment

1   Clearly, the House of Lords Select Committee found a considerable dispute between the Faculty and the Society of Homoeopaths. The Faculty's key concern seems to be that a shared core curriculum is irrelevant to them because the people they train are not the same as those the Society trains. In particular, they consider that orthodox health care staff already have a base of understanding, which includes subjects such as anatomy and physiology. Second, there is the issue of what kind of cases the Faculty's students will treat after graduation. The Faculty argues that medically trained homeopaths may end up working in a homeopathic hospital where both orthodox and homeopathic treatments are used. Therefore, a core curriculum should cover this kind of 'integrated' working to be useful to their graduates.

2   The Society argues that much needs to be learned beyond orthodox health care in order to become a homeopath. Arguably, there is an implication that the Society's approved curriculum conveys homeopathy in a way they consider to be more appropriate. It all seems to boil down to what each group believes a homeopath really needs to know.

Divisions between the Faculty and the Society of Homoeopaths have meant that the move towards regulation within homeopathy has been slow and difficult. As noted in Box 5.2, National Occupational Standards in the modality have been established but the Faculty (although involved in their development) has failed to use them in its own training.

5.4   Evidence and doubt in homeopathy

Advocates of homeopathy have in the past and continue now to seek social and scientific respectability, setting up colleges and establishing homeopathy to the extent that the House of Lords report (2000) defines it as one of the 'Big Five' CAM modalities. However, despite its presence in the NHS and its public popularity, there remains scientific scepticism about the modality and how or whether it works. Within medicine and science, there is as much powerful strength of feeling against homeopathy as there is for it, although the notion of a 'neutral, scientific procedure' that might be used objectively to determine the effectiveness of homeopathy can be, and has been, contested. Instead, 'scientific knowledge' may be considered as a socially constructed interpretation of the world, involving collective agreements among scientists about the meaning of phenomena and how to apply general rules of knowledge evaluation in particular circumstances. In short, it is possible to consider a process involving the social construction of knowledge about complementary therapy motivated by political and professional interests.

The history of homeopathy has given people who study the nature of science some interesting examples of how vehemently conventional science defends its own theories against evidence that might damage its credibility.

Supposedly objective scientific 'rules' for interpreting evidence – such as theoretical consistency with established knowledge and adequacy of experimental design – have been used creatively to preserve established boundaries between what is regarded as 'legitimate' and 'illegitimate' knowledge. The following case study is about the work of a French scientist, Dr Jacques Benveniste. It shows how the tactic was deployed of undermining the credibility of experimental results by impugning the character of the researchers, by suggesting fraud, and by dismissing experimentally adequate results because they are inconsistent with established knowledge.

THE CASE OF DR JACQUES BENVENISTE

Dr Benveniste and his associates apparently showed in experimental work that a certain type of white blood cell could be provoked into releasing histamine when exposed to levels of antibody in high homeopathic dilution. The paper detailing the work was published in the journal *Nature* (Davenas et al., 1988). The research had been extensively refereed, which failed to identify any crucial weakness in design or control. However, against convention, the editors of *Nature* only allowed the paper to be published with an editorial reservation which expressed 'incredulity', the opinion that there was 'no physical basis for such an activity', and an indication that arrangements had been made 'for independent investigators to observe repetition of the experiments' (Nature, 1988, p. 787). Note that it is not common practice for works submitted by esteemed scientists to be challenged in this way. The only difference in this research was that it appeared to support the idea that homeopathy could work and had worked in the experiments done by Benveniste's team.

The independent team of investigators comprised James Randi (a US-based magician and fraud-buster), Walter Stuart (a specialist in the study of misconduct in science) and John Maddox (a scientific journalist). They reported almost exactly a month later (Maddox et al., 1988). As far as they were concerned, the Benveniste experiments were 'statistically ill-controlled, from which no substantial effort has been made to exclude systematic error, including observer bias' and that 'the phenomenon described is not reproducible in the ordinary meaning of that word.' The implication of these remarks, in conjunction with the composition of the investigating team, was that the results could only be reproduced by trickery and self-delusion. Dr Benveniste, at first hailed as breaking new ground in scientific discovery, next found his work described as unscientific and his team of researchers as possible tricksters. His career was ruined and his laboratories closed down shortly afterwards. What is interesting in this case is that the lack of trust is not apparent in other areas of science. In other words, if a scientist submits a paper to an esteemed science journal generally it is most unlikely that a team will be sent to 'check out' the conditions under which the research took place or the skills of the researchers. The Benveniste case has meant that homeopathic research is under much greater scrutiny than other areas of science.

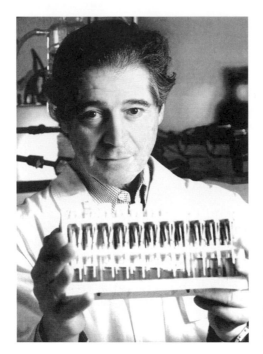

Jacques Benveniste — homeopath and researcher, attacked by the scientific establishment

The Benveniste case also illustrates the lack of trust shown by scientists who attempt to study the efficacy of CAM treatments. An example of this is a study made for the BBC television programme *Horizon* that was called 'Homoeopathy: The Test' (Randi, 2002). It was set up as a challenge and presented as a definitive test of whether or not homeopathy worked. Not only did it draw widespread media coverage but also it seemed to suggest that it could answer the questions posed by the Benveniste case. In the test all patients were treated the same by a single remedy being given to subjects suffering from allergies. It was a randomised controlled trial (RCT), as patients were given either the remedy or a placebo. It was also a double-blind test, as neither patients nor researchers knew who was given what. At the end the results were analysed by a separate group of researchers. The test appeared to be scientific and carefully organised so that no one person could affect the results.

James Randi featured on the programme and in the test in two ways: first, as a fraud-buster in science and, second, by offering a $1 million reward for proof of any kind of paranormal (unexplainable by science) phenomena. In this way, his input allowed the programme makers to bring in the twist of monetary reward for the success of the experiment. Randi's view is that homeopathy often involves the wishful thinking of the practitioner and the patient. He argues that the wish to believe is as powerful in science as anywhere else: 'scientists are human beings. Like anyone else they can fool themselves' (Randi, 2004). Randi was shown not only 'doing science' in the documentary (that is, gathering and seriously considering evidence) but also performing magic tricks.

The methodological problems in studying homeopathy were not explained in the programme and the ways in which the trial might be flawed were glossed over. To the general public this might have seemed like a fair test but you may have some doubts after reading about the way homeopathy is practised.

ACTIVITY   WAS THE *HORIZON* PROGRAMME A FAIR TEST OF HOMEOPATHY?

Allow 15 minutes

Do you think, from the account given above, that the homeopathy test was done fairly? Given the basic principles of the modality outlined in this chapter, can you see any problems with how the test was organised and what it set out to achieve? Base your response on whether you think it reflected the way homeopathy is practised rather than the more technical matters of research methodology.

Comment

It could be argued that there is a flaw in the *Horizon* study. It was a single remedy study. Practitioners would argue that such studies do not represent the way in which homeopathy is practised. Each remedy is chosen for an individual (not for a particular disease or illness), after a long consultation which aims to build up 'symptom pictures'. Homeopathy also operates with the notion of 'layers of illness', so a single remedy is inappropriate. Individual factors, such as character and personality, also affect the choice of treatment, which was not the case in the *Horizon* experiment, so it cannot be said to be a test of homeopathy.

The *Horizon* programme was interested in two aspects: not only testing homeopathy but also providing entertainment. The use of magic tricks and gimmicks suggests a less than serious and 'scientific' attitude to an important subject that affects many people.

What counts as adequate evidence is not a simple unambiguous matter of observation, or facts, or replicability, but a matter of a socially located point of view. Political processes will always, therefore, remain crucial areas of study in understanding the shifting boundaries between CAM and orthodox science.

However, the important question remains: does homeopathy work? It is very difficult to answer at this stage. Many orthodox practitioners and scientists would say no. This answer may come from the view that homeopathy cannot possibly work because of the lack of active ingredients in the remedies. However, there are many perspectives on the efficacy of homeopathy and, as with other CAM modalities, claims of success are often made by individual users or practitioners who have experienced good results for themselves. While such anecdotal evidence is important to those particular individuals, larger scale studies are needed to demonstrate whether specific CAM remedies work and are safe. There is a review of the research evidence base for homeopathy in Box 5.3.

BOX 5.3   THE RESEARCH EVIDENCE BASE FOR HOMEOPATHY

Fifty papers report a significant benefit of homeopathy in at least one clinical outcome measure, 41 that fail to discern any inter-group differences, and two that describe an inferior response with homeopathy. Considering the relative number of research articles on the 35 different medical conditions in which such research has been carried out, the weight of evidence currently favours a positive treatment effect in eight: childhood diarrhoea, fibrositis, hayfever, influenza, pain (miscellaneous), side-effects of radio- or chemotherapy, sprains and upper respiratory tract infection. Based on published research to date, it seems unlikely that homeopathy is efficacious for headache, stroke or warts. Insufficient research prevents conclusions from being drawn about any other medical conditions.

(Source: Mathie, 2003, p. 84)

Most research on homeopathy has taken the form of placebo-controlled RCTs of a single remedy, such as the one conducted for the *Horizon* programme. Some people are given a genuine homeopathic remedy, while others are given a placebo (fake pill). In this type of study a single remedy, such as arnica 6C, is used. It is important to note that, in real treatment, arnica 6C would not be given to two people with the same symptoms. The choice of remedy would be more sophisticated, involving a range of factors concerning the individual and their experience of the symptoms. RCTs often test one type of illness or disease, so they might test the effect of arnica C on delayed muscle soreness (after exercise, for example). Here again there is a problem between homeopathic treatment and such a study. Homeopaths do not treat just muscle pain: they use a remedy to treat a particular symptom picture. It is also important to remember that homeopathic treatment is often long and complex and involves changing remedies as the homeopath notes changes in the symptom pathway or picture. Therefore, RCTs are often not representative of actual treatment and how homeopaths work with patients. Chapter 7 explores this issue further and makes the case for more small-scale qualitative and longitudinal studies in CAM.

The University of York's NHS Centre for Reviews and Dissemination showed that major reviews of studies found there were such inconsistencies and difficulties in the quality of research into homeopathy that conclusions about efficacy could not be drawn:

> The evidence base for homeopathy needs to be interpreted with caution. Many of the areas that have been researched are not representative of the conditions that homeopathic practitioners usually treat. Additionally, all

conclusions about effectiveness should be considered together with the methodological problems of the research.

(Centre for Reviews and Dissemination, 2002, p. 1)

Other findings have been unequivocally negative. However, the problem of how to test homeopathy for efficacy remains. Homeopaths are unlikely to accept findings based on single-remedy studies. There is a greater call for studies to look at outcome and at the experience of individuals throughout the course of their treatment. This could mean following someone for a year or even longer. It remains to be seen whether orthodox science will take up the challenge and study homeopathy on its own terms.

Regulating homeopathic preparations: can the imperceptible be regulated?

It is not only the world of science that is affected by the problems of trying to understand how homeopathy could work. As homeopathy is so popular – both over the counter and in face-to-face consultations with a practitioner – there are also issues about regulating the manufacture of homeopathic medicines. This is important to ensure both that homeopathic preparations are safe and that claims made on medicines are accurate and represent value for money. In essence, the user of homeopathic medicines is a consumer and expects to be protected from dangerous and fraudulent practice. However, homeopaths are in a difficult position when it comes to fraudulence. As a scientific anomaly – that is a set of practices that do not fit with conventional scientific principles and explanations – homeopathy is in a poor position to fight its corner with research-based claims of efficacy. As shown above, there is little agreement within the scientific community on whether homeopathy can or does work, and studies that seem to show it working have often been inadequately carried out. Disputes between proponents and opponents over how homeopathy can be scientifically tested add to the difficulties of separating fraud from useful treatments. This leads to the interesting dilemma of how regulators and licensers of the pharmaceutical market should treat homeopathic medicines.

In the UK, the Medicines and Healthcare products Regulatory Agency (MHRA) regulates medicines and is responsible for protecting public health by maintaining standards of safety, quality and efficacy. However, homeopathic medicines are difficult because, on the one hand, the law of dilution should mean there is little active ingredient (thus no chance of injury from overdose or misuse) and, on the other hand, manufacturers and practitioners alike maintain that they are potent drugs. In the UK, the MHRA does not treat homeopathic drugs in the same way as other drugs, whether orthodox or herbal medicines. The Medicines Act 1971 grants licences for the homeopathic remedies existing at that time to be manufactured and sold. However, after 1971 all new remedies had to pass stringent conventional clinical trials (the same as any other drug). A European Directive (92/73 EEC) later allowed a slimline process of registration of homeopathic drugs in the UK:

> In order to qualify for registration the products must:
>
> ■ be for oral or external use. This includes all methods of administration with the exception of injections;
>
> ■ be sufficiently dilute to guarantee their safety;
>
> ■ make no therapeutic claims.

So, there is a trade-off in that registration means that no claims can be made about the efficacy of homeopathic medicines (MHRA, 2003).

The situation is similar in the USA, where the Food and Drug Administration (FDA) is responsible for regulating homeopathic medicines. Stehlin (1996) notes that homeopathic products are exempt from goods-manufacturing requirements that relate to product testing for the strength of active ingredients and expiry date testing. The drugs only need an imprint identifying the manufacturer and that the drug is homeopathic but nothing to indicate which remedy it is. Homeopathic drugs are also allowed to contain more alcohol than orthodox ones, as it is considered a traditional ingredient of these remedies. Again there is an issue of trying to regulate a group of 'drugs' that in terms of chemical constitution are nothing more than sugar pills. The irony has not been lost on fraud-busting groups who demand that all health care and medical products are tested on a scientific basis. In the USA, one such group is HomeoWatch, a similar group to QuackWatch, but focusing especially on homeopathy. Such groups view the differential treatment of homeopathic remedies as damaging to consumers, in terms of both their health and their pockets:

> The marketing of homeopathic products and services fits the definition of quackery established by a United States House of Representatives committee which investigated the problem (i.e., the promotion of 'medical schemes or remedies known to be false, or which are unproven, for a profit'). The United States Food, Drug, and Cosmetic Act lists the Homeopathic Pharmacopeia of the United States as a recognized compendium, but this status was due to political influence, not scientific merit. The FDA has not required homeopathic products to meet the efficacy requirements applied to all other drugs, creating an unacceptable double standard for drug marketing.
>
> (National Council Against Health Fraud, 1993, p. 2)

For groups such as the NCAHF, homeopathy is a misguided form of medicine and the lack of scientific back-up is only the starting point for a critique of its spread and success.

Although the issue of whether or how homeopathic remedies 'work' is a major bone of contention for medical scientists, the fact that they perceive that the remedies do work makes it attractive to many orthodox medical practitioners. They are less concerned about whether it violates the laws of physics, and more interested in being able to give an option to patients for whom biomedicine offers little, especially one without unwanted side effects (May and Sirur, 1988).

5.5   Conclusion

This chapter focused on homeopathy to put the issues developed in Chapters 1 to 4 into a particular context. The basic principles of homeopathy developed by Hahnemann were explained and the ways homeopathic knowledge and its status have changed since its inception were explored. The chapter documented how these basic principles and the knowledge base of homeopathy have been constantly challenged and accusations of fraud made. Nevertheless, a great deal of trust has been put in homeopathy, not only by users but also by qualified medical practitioners. Homeopathy is thus a fascinating example of a CAM modality which, despite being considered scientifically incredible, has managed to gain much public acceptance as well as some level of medical support. It is available on the NHS and is practised by a sizeable proportion of medical practitioners. However, this has led to some problems. In effect, a dual profession has emerged, causing difficulties for the education and training of practitioners, especially in terms of establishing an appropriate curriculum. Similarly, the question of regulation and control is problematic with one strand of practitioners being highly regulated and the others not.

In some situations the practice of homeopathy is considered a threat to orthodox, 'scientific' concepts of health and has attracted a vehement backlash from within the medical and scientific communities. However, the principles of homeopathy developed by Hahnemann remain irrepressibly popular.

KEY POINTS

- ■ Homeopathy remains a popular form of CAM. Increasing numbers of people use over-the-counter homeopathy or consult homeopathic practitioners.

- ■ Growing numbers of medical professionals are involved in the study and practice of homeopathy, even though they have been trained in orthodox medicine.

- ■ Homeopathy has always enjoyed the patronage of certain rich and famous adherents, including members of the Royal Family who have bestowed the title 'Royal' on several British homeopathic hospitals.

- ■ The basic tenets of homeopathy are diametrically opposed to the principles underlying orthodox medical practice.

- ■ The history of homeopathy includes many instances of the medical and scientific establishments attacking its practice.

- ■ Each homeopathic remedy is individually tailored to the individual person attending for treatment, so it is hard to carry out randomised controlled trials and other scientific tests of efficacy.

- ■ Although many research trials have found evidence of the effectiveness of homeopathic remedies, the jury is still out regarding how it works or whether much of the positive effect perceived by users is caused by the placebo effect.

References

Castro, M. (1990) *The Complete Homeopathy Handbook*, London, Macmillan.

Centre for Reviews and Dissemination (2002) 'Homeopathy', *Effective Health Care*, Vol. 7, No. 3, pp. 1–12. Available online at: www.york.ac.uk/inst/crd/ehc73.pdf [accessed 25 September 2004].

Cullen, W. (1789) *Treatise of the Materia Medica*, London, T. Lowndes.

Davenas, E., Beauvais, F., Arnara, J., Oberbaum, M., Robinson, B., Miadonna, A., Tedeschi, A., Pomeranz, B., Fortner, P., Belon, P., Sainte-Laudy, J., Poitevin, B. and Benveniste, J. (1988) 'Human basophil degranulation triggered by very dilute antiserum against IgE', *Nature*, Vol. 333, No. 6176, pp. 816–18.

Hahnemann, S. (1810) *Organon der Rationellen Heilkunde* (*The Organon of Rational Healing*), Dresden, Arnold.

Hardy, J. (2003) *Bird Remedies* [online], www.marlev.com/homeo/Study%20Room/Library/LibraryBirds.htm [accessed 29 November 2004].

House of Lords (2000) Select Committee on Science and Technology's Sixth Report, *Complementary and Alternative Medicine*, London, The Stationery Office. Available online at: www.publications.parliament.uk/pa/ld199900/ldselect/ldsctech/123/1234.htm [accessed 29 November 2004].

Jonas, W. B., Kaptchuk, T. J. and Linde, K. (2003) 'A critical overview of homeopathy', *Annals of Internal Medicine*, Vol. 138, No. 5, pp. 393–9.

Maddox, J., Randi, J. and Stewart, W. (1988) '"High-dilution" experiments a delusion', *Nature*, Vol. 334, No. 6180, p. 287.

Mathie, R. T. (2003) 'The research evidence base for homeopathy: a fresh assessment of the literature', *Homeopathy*, Vol. 92, No. 2, pp. 84–91.

(May, C. and Sirur, D., 1988) 'Art, science and placebo', *Sociology of Health and Illness*, Vol. 20, No. 2, pp. 168–90.

Medicines and Healthcare products Regulatory Agency (2003) *The Control and Quality of Homeopathic Stocks*, London, MHRA.

National Council Against Health Fraud (1993) *Position Paper on Homeopathy* [online], www.ncahf.org/pp/homeop.html [accessed 29 November 2004].

Nature (1988) Editorial: 'When to believe the unbelievable', *Nature*, Vol. 333, No. 6176, p. 787.

Porter, R. (1999) *The Greatest Benefit to Mankind: A Medical History of Humanity from Antiquity to the Present*, London, Fontana Press.

Randi, J. (2002) *Homoeopathy: The Test*, programme summary [online], www.bbc.co.uk/science/horizon/2002/homeopathy.shtml [accessed 25 September 2004].

Scott, A. (1998) 'Homeopathy as a feminist form of medicine', *Sociology of Health and Illness*, Vol. 20, No. 2, pp. 191–214.

Stehlin, I. (1996) 'Homeopathy: real medicine or empty promises?', *FDA Consumer Magazine*, December. Available online at: www.fda.gov/fdac/features/096_home.html [accessed 25 September 2004].

World Health Organization (WHO) (2004) *The WHO Strategy for Traditional Medicine* [online], www.emro.who.int/rc49/document_49/3.htm [accessed 16 February 2005].

Researching Complementary and Alternative Medicine

Edited by Tom Heller and Hilary MacQueen

Chapter 6 A critical look at orthodox medical approaches

Tom Heller, Dick Heller and Gavin Yamey

Contents

AIMS

- To discuss the ways in which research and evidence can illustrate the practice of orthodox medicine.
- To evaluate the key factors underpinning the debate about evidence-based medicine.
- To introduce the issues around the placebo effect and how it relates to CAM therapies.

6.1 Introduction

This book and its companion volume take a critical look at complementary and alternative medicine (CAM). It has explored a wide range of issues about the use and misuse of CAM and promoted an understanding of the place in contemporary society of this approach to health and illness. It is now time for orthodox medical approaches to be similarly scrutinised. This chapter explores various aspects of orthodox (or allopathic, modern or western) medicine and will help you to understand further perspectives on how it has developed and the role that it now plays. This chapter will not make orthodox approaches seem in competition or in conflict with complementary and alternative forms of practice; rather, it will help you understand more about this subject area so that you can form your own view of the relationship between various health care systems and practices.

6.2   What's in a name?

The way in which different systems and approaches to health care are named and labelled can reveal interesting, and perhaps important, insights into the philosophies underlying their practice. The use of the terms 'alternative' and 'complementary' is heavily debated. In a sociological sense these terms signal their relationship to the dominant health care system: as outsiders. CAM is put firmly in its place by designating and defining its philosophies and practices in relation to 'mainstream' or prevailing medical practice. CAM therapies remain outside, 'alternative' or, at best, somehow achieve the status of 'complementary handmaidens'. However, the labels that are attached to the predominant health care system can also be revealing. Some people use the word 'allopathic', which emerged relatively recently (in the 19th century) as a label for the system that uses remedies that are different from, or opposed to, the presenting complaint. This definition was probably introduced by homeopaths, to distinguish it from their approach, which treats complaints with remedies that produce similar symptoms to the condition being treated. The dominant medical system is also sometimes labelled 'western' medicine, to distinguish it from 'traditional' medicine, which the World Health

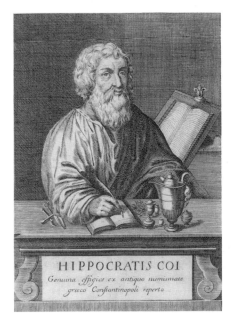

Since the time of Hippocrates (400 BC) there has been tension between empiricists, who went on to become holistic and naturopathic healers, and rationalists, who are today's scientific doctors

Organization and others define in relation to the cultural norms of the country in which it is practised (WHO, 2003).

Perhaps most interesting of all, there is the term 'scientific medicine'. The history of this concept can be traced back to two distinct medical systems that were part of separate philosophical approaches from the time of the Greek 'father of medicine' Hippocrates (400 BC). One strand was known as the **empiricist**, or 'vitalist', approach and this developed into the **holistic** and **naturopathic** traditions. The other strand, which developed into the **scientific** approach, was known as the **rationalist** approach. The original debate centred on one question: 'Which is the more appropriate way to obtain truth and knowledge: through experience (the vitalists) or through reasoning (the rationalists)?' It is possible to trace the way in which current philosophical debates between CAM and 'scientific' medicine have evolved from this central divergence of opinion. Indeed, the 'scientific defence' that emanates from the currently dominant medical establishment, and which attempts to keep CAM modalities in their place, could not be clearer:

> What most sets alternative medicine apart, in our view, is that it has not been scientifically tested and its advocates largely deny the need for such testing. By testing we mean the marshaling of rigorous evidence of safety and efficacy ... Of course, many treatments used in conventional medicine have not been rigorously tested, either, but the scientific community generally acknowledges that this is a failing that needs to be remedied.
>
> (Angell and Kassirer, 1998, p. 839)

The dominant medical system uses a variety of 'scientific' approaches to understand and combat disease. In many ways this approach has been enormously effective. Many major health problems have been subjected to intense, systematic scrutiny and there are plenty of examples of diseases that have been 'conquered', and where levels of understanding have reached great heights. However, the system also has costs, sometimes at the expense of the approaches that are now called 'alternative', or that cannot claim the resources or societal approval that mainstream medicine attracts. Precisely because of the importance of this medical endeavour, it is also imperative to look critically at its achievements, which is the subject of this chapter.

A certain type of language is used to describe orthodox approaches to health and healing. The words used often seem to be combative and involve terms associated with 'battles', 'struggles' and 'fights' against disease. In everyday speech, and certainly in the media, phrases such as 'Jamie lost his battle with cancer' or 'New drug introduced to fight arthritis' are common. This language, and the metaphors and images that are conjured up, do seem to shed light on how practitioners of orthodox medicine set about their task, which is in stark contrast to many of the concepts and philosophical ideas associated with complementary and alternative therapies.

The logic of orthodox medicine

The 'scientific' approach to 'conquering' disease could be characterised as a reductionist task that can be split into a series of logical steps. First, the cause of the disease is identified: for example, the bacillus (or germ) that causes pneumonia. The next step involves understanding how the bacillus works within the host organism, followed by the development of an agent that will eliminate or kill the bacillus. No wonder war-like imagery has developed alongside orthodox medicine to describe its 'advances' and 'victories'. Many categories of medication have adopted a nomenclature that seems to illustrate this combative feature that is inherent in many modern pharmaceutical products. For example, the British National Formulary (2004), which lists all medical products licensed for use on humans, has many entries with 'anti-' in their title: anti-acne, anti-allergy, anti-androgen, anti-anginal, anti-arrythmic, anti-asthma, etc.

6.3   The cornerstones of contemporary medical practice

Over several centuries, and in many countries, a concerted effort has been made to understand anatomy, physiology and pathology. This has allowed medical practice to develop in a way that can legitimately be called 'scientific'. Before the English physician William Harvey (1578–1657) published *An Anatomical Study of the Motion of the Heart and of the Blood in Animals* in 1628, it was not known how blood circulates around the body. This realisation could only result from the development of the scientific method, for which it is necessary to thank Sir Francis Bacon (1561–1626), who suggested that reason rather than faith should underlie knowledge (Bacon, 1605). This idea developed during the Elizabethan period (1558–1603), which was also a time of growth in industry, commerce and art. This Elizabethan Renaissance, together with the Italian Renaissance, was the beginning of the modern European world.

Similarly, the cause of infections was obscure before the French chemist and bacteriologist Louis Pasteur (1822–1895) worked on human infectious diseases from 1875 to 1887. During the 19th and 20th centuries, the basic understanding of normal functioning and of the patterns and causes of many diseases grew enormously. The causes of different types of infectious disease were identified: for example, the organism responsible for tuberculosis (TB) was identified in 1882 by the German bacteriologist Robert Koch (1843–1910). From the mid-20th century, when antibiotics were first discovered, physicians could provide effective treatment for some types of infection. Diseases such as TB, which had previously killed so many people, could be treated successfully through the further application of the scientific method. Many of the previous attempts at sometimes heroic treatments for TB – such

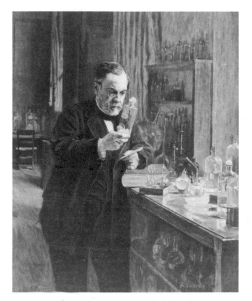

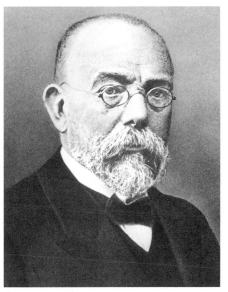

Before the work of Louis Pasteur, the cause of infections was not understood

Robert Koch discovered the cause of tuberculosis

as long periods of incarceration in a sanatorium in the mountains – which had neither been based on a scientific rationale nor subjected to scientific evaluation of their benefits, could then be abandoned.

ACTIVITY   ORTHODOX MEDICAL SUCCESSES AND TRIUMPHS

Allow 20 minutes

What do you think are the greatest advances in medical science and why?

You could also ask some of your friends and family. You may have a personal reason or significant experience for regarding a particular scientific medical advance as being important.

Comment

People who did this activity thought of many medical treatments and procedures that were particularly significant. As anticipated, there were often personal reasons for some of their choices, for example:

'The discovery of insulin and other modern treatments for diabetes — because my middle daughter has diabetes and wouldn't have survived without these advances.'

'Coronary artery bypass surgery — my father has had an extra few years of life because of the operation.'

'Kidney dialysis — the young lad who lives across the road has a machine in his bedroom now and he has got another chance to live until he gets a transplant.'

Renal failure: an example of orthodox scientific medicine in practice

The kidneys' function is to rid the body of the unwanted by-products of metabolism. Without working kidneys there would be a fatal build-up of metabolic products in the body. A (biochemical) marker of this build-up is creatinine, which is a breakdown product of muscle. Increased blood levels of creatinine indicate deteriorating kidney (or renal) function. It was not until the second half of the 20th century that scientific experimental inquiry led to the development of artificial ways to remove waste products such as creatinine from the body: renal dialysis was born. Using techniques developed in the experimental laboratory, the patient's blood could now be passed over specially produced, semi-permeable membranes and the waste products filtered out. This is obviously a very shorthand way of describing a major technical advance! Later it was discovered that it was possible to surgically replace a kidney. The main problem with this procedure is that placing the kidney of another person (either a living relative or someone who has recently died) into a person with renal failure could trigger a reaction – an immune response – when the body recognises the new kidney as being foreign. In turn, this causes the new kidney to be rejected and stop working. However, the developing science of immunology led to the identification of drugs that could largely prevent this immunological rejection.

Of course, an even better way of helping the problem of renal failure is to prevent it happening in the first place. Epidemiologists have identified many of the major causes of kidney failure in humans. These vary according to the population and, within any population, according to several factors. Untreated or poorly treated high blood pressure used to be a major cause but, as medical detection and care improve, this is now less common – a major success for preventive medicine. Kidney failure can also result from urinary tract infection, and the recognition and prevention of this has also been a major advance. The progression of the disease can be slowed once it has become established and several interventions may help, such as various dietary restrictions.

6.4 Evidence-based medicine

The understanding of disease mechanisms and the availability of diagnostic testing and treatments are not sufficient to ensure that the best diagnosis is made and the most appropriate treatment is given. The problem is that probability is always involved, which surprisingly large numbers of health professionals do not appreciate. There are no absolutely certain diagnostic tests or procedures. A particular result found in the laboratory only reflects the degree of probability of a disease being present in the person who produced the sample. A treatment based on sound physiological principles may or may not result in real benefit to people with the disease. A treatment that appears to work when given to one particular person may not work in other people. The discipline of **evidence-based medicine** (EBM), and its various extensions to non-medical health care activities, was developed in an attempt to introduce a scientific basis to health care practice. EBM has been defined as a basic science for clinical practice (Sackett et al., 1996). It has now been extended to all the health care professions within orthodox medicine and it involves both 'statistical' and 'implementation' aspects (Heller and Page, 2002).

One statistical approach is the science of reviewing all the published research studies of a particular condition. This methodology is called **systematic review** and various statistical methods, such as **meta-analysis**, are used to analyse these collections of results. The Cochrane Collaboration (2004) collects and publishes such reviews and analyses, and makes them available on the internet, including complementary and alternative treatments that have been subjected to this approach. Most of the studies that are reviewed are **randomised controlled trials** (RCTs). The first of these, and in many ways the basis of techniques that evolved into EBM, was a trial of the use of streptomycin to treat TB in 1948, which was published in the *British Medical Journal* (Medical Research Council, 1948). This research was necessary because initially only limited supplies of streptomycin were available. The benefits associated with the new antibiotic were numerous and readily uncovered using these investigative techniques.

The term 'evidence-based medicine' was first used in the late 1980s by a group of clinical epidemiologists at McMaster University in Canada, who defined it as:

> the conscientious, explicit, and judicious use of current best evidence in making decisions about the care of individual patients. The practice of evidence based medicine means integrating individual clinical expertise with the best available external clinical evidence from systematic research.
>
> (Sackett et al., 1996, p. 71)

At its heart, then, the practice of EBM requires health professionals to make decisions about treatment that are based on the best evidence available from a search of all the literature. This immediately raises some obstacles to practising EBM. For example, how would a busy, inner-city general practitioner (GP) find time to search the entire literature?

The concept of 'best evidence' is central to EBM because it has a hierarchy of what it considers 'good evidence' and 'bad evidence'. In EBM the best evidence of whether a particular treatment works comes from synthesising the results of all well designed RCTs of that treatment. The weakest evidence is opinion ('It works because I say it works'), anecdote ('It works because we've heard that it works') and case study ('It's bound to work on everyone because it helped Mrs Jones'). Practitioners of EBM always try to use the best available evidence in making decisions about treatment.

Why was EBM such a new idea? After all, what were doctors doing before EBM? Surely they read about research findings and applied them to their practice? In reality, before EBM, doctors generally combined their clinical experience, their knowledge of basic disease mechanisms, and the research results they might have seen in the latest *British Medical Journal*. What was missing was systematic access to **all** of the **best quality** research evidence that doctors could then apply to the care of **all** their patients.

The limitations of EBM

In many ways, EBM had an enthusiastic reception among health professionals – from clinicians through to policy makers. The original concept of EBM led to an explosion of new journals, such as *Evidence-Based Nursing* and *Evidence-Based Mental Health*, which were dedicated to evidence-based practice. Academic centres for the promotion of EBM sprang up around the world, and committed themselves to promoting, among other subjects, evidence-based adult medicine, child health, surgery, pathology, pharmacotherapy, nursing, general practice and dentistry.

ACTIVITY   BENEFITS OF AND CONCERNS ABOUT EBM

Allow 15 minutes

Think about the concept of EBM and how health service professionals, already working to their limits, might have greeted its arrival.

■ What benefits might the professionals have envisaged?

■ What concerns might they have had about EBM and its implementation?

Comment

People who did this activity thought that professionals might have the following concerns, which are considered further in the rest of this section.

■ There are major practical barriers to using EBM — we just do not have enough time to study the evidence.

■ EBM can only answer certain questions — people and their problems are usually more complex.

■ EBM gives no information about patients in the real world. It is all based on trials that do not necessarily reflect clinical reality. In any case, the pharmaceutical industry drives the evidence behind EBM.

■ EBM advocates 'cookbook medicine' — it removes professional autonomy and patient individuality and has the tone of a moral crusade.

Concerns about implementing EBM

EBM has had its fair share of detractors, who point to moral, ethical, ideological and practical barriers to using it. There are major practical barriers to using EBM. There are too few support structures to help professionals find and appraise the research literature that can guide them in practising EBM. Furthermore, when professionals do look for evidence on a particular health topic, they often do not find any.

In theory at least, EBM can answer only certain questions, such as 'What is the chance that X benefits or harms people?', where X includes a medication, an operation or any other intervention in people's health. EBM cannot answer 'How?' or 'Why?' questions about how the world works or how people are feeling (Donald, 2002). So, EBM is helpful for deciding whether to carry out certain procedures (for example, RCTs to help decide whether healthy men should be screened for prostate cancer) but it is not so helpful for finding out how a patient feels or why a particular disease behaves in the way it does.

EBM gives no information about people who are in the real world. Remember, the 'best' evidence in EBM comes from RCTs. In these trials, a treatment is tested on people under strict study conditions. There are often very strict inclusion criteria determining which people can enter the trial. This means it can be difficult to apply the trial results to the people who attend a clinic because they may be very different from the people tested in the trial.

For example, an important new study shows that a new drug, X, helps people with angina (chest pain from coronary artery disease). A GP reads about the study in the *British Medical Journal* and sees that it is well designed and that the results are reliable. The GP is excited because there are many people on the practice list with angina who might benefit from being given drug X. But then the GP reads the study more closely. People who were over 65, who smoked, or had high cholesterol or diabetes were excluded from the study. So, what does the GP do about Mr Jones, who has angina but is 68, smokes and has diabetes? Will drug X work for him? EBM is almost certainly **not** helpful when it comes to treating Mr Jones.

The pharmaceutical industry also drives the evidence behind EBM. One of the biggest problems with EBM is that many (perhaps most) of the trials on which it is based have been funded by industry (Choudhury et al., 2002). This is problematic because studies funded by drug companies are more likely to produce results that are favourable to these companies than studies funded through other sources (Abraham, 2002; Lexchin et al., 2003). In other words, the 'evidence' behind EBM is arguably driven by the vested interests of the pharmaceutical industry (Moynihan, 2003; Prosser et al., 2003). In particular, industry is generally only interested in funding trials that will help it to market new drugs. So, there are too few trials addressing issues that might be of major importance to patients that will also be profitable to the industry (for example, whether changing diet would help prevent disease).

EBM could be thought to advocate 'cookbook medicine' – it removes professional autonomy and the individuality of the people who attend for treatment. This is one of the most commonly cited criticisms of EBM. The argument here is that EBM is almost dictating how people with problems should be treated, as if doctors in particular should follow a formula or an algorithm. There is a risk that EBM could denigrate professionals' clinical expertise and ignore individuals' preferences and ideals.

Some commentators claim that EBM has the tone of a moral crusade. It can be argued that EBM has no particular moral stance: that it is just a way of answering certain clinical questions (Donald, 2002). However, advocates of EBM believe that clinicians 'ought to be responsible for keeping up to date with these advances and ought to be prepared to offer them to patients' (Haynes, 2002, p. 3). In this sense, EBM **does** have the flavour of a moral crusade.

Ironically, there is no evidence that practising EBM leads to a healthier population. In other words, there are simply no high-quality studies showing that people whose doctors practise EBM are better off than people whose doctors do not.

6.5 Why evidence does not always change medical practice

One of the greatest challenges facing advocates of EBM is that medical professionals seem extremely resistant to change. For example, important life-saving new treatments are only slowly disseminated into practice (Mair et al., 1996; Mashru and Lant, 1997; Sudlow et al., 1997), while practitioners are slow to abandon treatments from their practice which have been shown to be useless (Antman et al., 1992).

For a start, clinicians are bombarded daily with information from new trials and from many different sources. Very few of these studies are directly relevant to their practice, and yet they are spread thinly throughout many medical publications.

Freeman and Sweeney (2001) interviewed GPs in south-west England. They wanted to find out why GPs sometimes followed evidence-based guidance when treating people and yet at other times departed from this guidance. They found that a complex interplay of factors affects the decision. For example, GPs who had seen that a particular evidence-based treatment worked were positive about recommending it. In addition, the GPs perceived a tension between what they could do in the real world of primary care and the more rigorous approach recommended by specialist clinics. There was also a feeling among GPs that it could be difficult to apply evidence-based treatments to individual people: it was as if the doctors were 'shaping the square peg of the evidence to fit the round hole of the patient's life' (Freeman and Sweeney, 2001, p. 1102).

At health policy level, changing practice requires change at several different levels – from the organisation to the individual. For example, doctors have long known that people having a heart attack are more likely to survive if they are given clot-busting drugs (thrombolytics) through a vein within an hour. However, many people are still not given this treatment in time (Doorey et al., 1992; Ketley and Woods, 1993). This is because sometimes people fail to recognise the symptoms of a heart attack, or there are delays in getting them to hospital in time, or they may not be seen immediately by a health professional who recognises the problem and initiates treatment. These are just some of the barriers to the implementation of life-saving treatment.

Individual and population-based approaches

When people become sick, it is difficult for them to think beyond their own wish to get better. In these personal situations, evidence-based medicine can be the first casualty. What if the resources used to treat one person mean that someone else cannot have the treatment they require? What if there are more serious or more common conditions that could be treated in the population? What if using all the resources required for one person's treatment means there is nothing left over for preventing illness in others? Should the approach of the individual person, and the advocacy of this by their doctor, take precedence over the needs of the wider community? How could a discussion of this issue be initiated in the public domain so that resources can be allocated in a way that most effectively meets the requirements of the population?

For example, consider the situation of a person who is discovered to have a partially blocked artery that carries blood to the brain (the carotid artery). Surgeons can unblock this artery and there is evidence from well conducted RCTs that this will reduce the chance of the individual having a stroke in subsequent years. The cost of this identification and surgery is between £16,000 and £86,000 for each year of life gained by the individual (Hitt, 2001). Is this cost acceptable to the National Health Service (NHS), which has to pay the bill? Another way of preventing stroke is to give aspirin to people who are at risk – the cost of this is £40 for each year of life gained by these people (Hitt, 2001). Individuals want to preserve their life and maintain their health without suffering the consequences of a stroke (which could leave them unable to speak and dependent on someone else for the activities of daily living). How can these two potential benefits be compared? How can this situation be compared with the costs of a kidney transplant?

The best treatment for a person who has a stroke is to use a thrombolytic drug to unblock the blocked artery. Only seven people have to be treated with such an agent to prevent one of those seven dying or becoming dependent on someone else. Using aspirin in this situation, 33 people have to be treated to prevent a bad outcome. It seems obvious that the decision should be to use the 'unblocker'. However, closer inspection of the data reveals that only 4 per cent of people who have a stroke are eligible for the treatment because (a) it is only effective if given very soon after the stroke and (b) it can only be used after a head scan to ensure it is not used for a type of stroke where it would cause more harm than good. Aspirin can be given to 70 per cent of people after a stroke. It is less beneficial to the individual but it can be used in more people and it costs much less (Ebrahim, 1999). The balance between benefits to the individual and the population is complex, is the basis of much health policy decision-making, and has led to a set of methods being developed to extend EBM by giving it a population focus (Heller and Dobson, 2000).

6.6   Powerful medicine and its side effects: an ill for every pill?

In this section some of the potential problems associated with the use of modern pharmaceutical agents are considered. Modern medicines are potentially enormously powerful. They are designed and produced specifically to change the way various bodily functions work and no part of the body or metabolic process has escaped the attentions of the protagonists who promote the pharmaceutical endeavour. Of course, if a person or someone close to them becomes ill, or one of their organs starts to malfunction, it seems 'only natural' to do everything possible to correct the problem. Individuals might consider that, if there is a 'scientific' solution to the deficiency, what is the problem with using the chemical remedy? Ivan Illich (1976) was one of the first researchers to question this approach. He suggests that modern medicine has become a threat to health by undermining the inherent capacity and capability of individuals, and indeed entire societies, to cope with inevitable pain, sickness and death. More recent commentators question the way in which medicine has apparently encroached on so many aspects of contemporary life:

> The bad things of life: old age, death, pain, and handicap are thrust on
> doctors to keep families and society from facing them. Some of them are an
> integral part of medicine, and accepted as such. But there is a boundary
> beyond which medicine has only a small role.
>
> (Leibovici and Lièvre, 2002, p. 866)

ACTIVITY   USING ORTHODOX MEDICINE

Allow 20 minutes

Think about an occasion when you used a prescribed pharmaceutical product. Perhaps you take medication regularly for a persistent condition or recently had an episode where medication was prescribed. If you have no recent experience of this, think of a time when someone you know used a form of medication.

■ What condition was the medication prescribed for?

■ What do you think might have happened if the medication had not been taken?

■ Do you believe that there were risks associated with taking the medication?

■ What was the outcome of taking the medication?

Comment

People who did this activity seem to be typical of members of the general public. Several of them were taking regular medication, for example for high blood pressure:

> 'I take four different tablets every morning. It's really just part of my routine. I know that these have helped to get my pressure down to normal and that this reduces my chances of having a heart attack or a stroke or kidney failure. They are powerful tablets and I certainly feel more tired since taking them. I do tend to panic if I go away on a trip and forget my tablets.'

Other people remembered taking medication for a specific episode but it was a bad experience:

> 'I took some new antibiotics that my doctor prescribed for a skin infection. It seemed to clear up the infected area, but I came out in a terrible rash all over my body and had to stop the tablets after three days. I still feel itchy when the weather is hot and I put it all down to those tablets.'

Individual medicines can cause problems and, of course, combinations of different tablets can be even more problematic, but what is the scale of the problem? In 2001, the Audit Commission estimated that in the UK approximately 11 per cent of patients on hospital medical wards experienced an 'adverse event', such as being given the wrong drug or having a bad reaction to a drug (see Figure 6.1 overleaf). The report estimated that such events, although mainly non-fatal, each led to an average additional stay in hospital of 8.5 days and cost the NHS as much as £1.1 billion each year in total (Audit Commission, 2001).

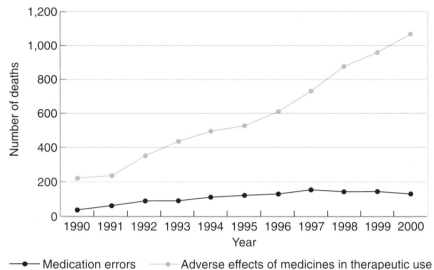

Figure 6.1   Number of deaths from medication errors and adverse effects of medicines, England and Wales, 1990–2000 (Source: Audit Commission, 2001, p. 19)

Vincent et al. (2001) studied adverse events in UK hospitals and found that they constituted a 'serious source of harm' (p. 517). They looked in detail at over 1000 medical records and found that the rates of adverse events vary between patients admitted under the care of different specialities (see Table 6.1 opposite), but there were potentially serious problems in all of them:

> About half of these [adverse] events were judged preventable. A third of adverse events led to moderate or greater disability or death. Some adverse events are serious and are traumatic for both staff and patients. Others are frequent, minor events that go unnoticed in routine clinical care and yet together have massive economic consequences.
>
> (Vincent et al., 2001, p. 518)

The apparently high level of problems associated with the use of powerful modern medicines has also been reported in the USA (Brennan et al., 1991) and Australia (Wilson et al., 1995). These studies, as well as the UK study by the Audit Commission, relied on reviews of the medical records of hospital admissions. Even more startling findings are reported from direct observation of what goes on at the bedside as the following quotation shows.

TABLE 6.1 NUMBER OF ADVERSE EVENTS BY SPECIALITY					
		No. of patients with adverse events detected		Total no. of adverse events detected	
Speciality	No. (%) of records reviewed	All (% of records)	Preventable (% of events)	All (% of records)	Preventable (% of events)
General medicine	273 (27)	24 (8.8)	18 (75)	25 (9.2)	19 (76)
General surgery	290 (29)	41 (14.1)	17 (41)	47 (16.2)	20 (43)
Obstetrics	174 (17)	7 (4.0)	5 (71)	7 (4.0)	5 (71)
Orthopaedics	277 (27)	38 (13.7)	12 (32)	40 (14.4)	13 (33)
Total	1014	110 (10.8)	52 (47)	119 (11.7)	57 (48)

(Source: Vincent et al., 2001, p. 518)

Observational studies, although costly, have identified even higher rates of error and injury occurring during medical care. For example, observers on the general surgical units of a Chicago teaching hospital who recorded all 'situations in which an inappropriate decision was made when, at the time, an appropriate alternative could have been chosen' found that 45.8% of patients experienced an adverse event [Andrews et al., 1997]. Eighteen per cent of these patients had a 'serious' adverse event – that is, one that produced at least temporary disability.

Similarly, Donchin et al. [1995] placed an observer at the patient's bedside to observe clinicians in the medical-surgical intensive care unit of a university hospital in Israel. Clinicians made 554 errors over four months, or 1.7 errors per patient per day.

(Weingart et al., 2000, p. 774)

There are many problems associated with attempts to determine precisely the extent of medical error and with using and prescribing medication. It can be difficult to determine whether a particular adverse effect is a property of the medication itself, or whether the health care system or individual workers within the service are at fault. Indeed, the whole notion of fault and blame has become a problem in itself (Berwick and Leape, 1999). Professionals are less likely to report, and subsequently learn from, any possible errors or 'near misses' that they might have been associated with, for fear of blame and punishment and, of course, the threat of potentially large legal settlements may not be far behind (Blendon et al., 2003).

ACTIVITY   ADVERSE EVENTS

Allow 20 minutes

What differences could there be between adverse events that occur within orthodox medical services (for example, with prescribed medication) and those that may occur in the practice of complementary and alternative approaches?

Comment

There are many potential problems both within the orthodox medical services, such as the NHS, and within the sphere of complementary and alternative health care. Most orthodox forms of medicine are practised within a health care structure. In the UK the majority of medical and health care practice is within the NHS, with a small but significant proportion in the private sector. All of this activity, and every action of registered medical practitioners, is tightly controlled by a series of Acts of Parliament and other legal and statutory regulatory devices. This means that if a service user feels aggrieved, or considers they have been damaged as a result of medical malpractice, or has a problem associated with the use or misuse of medication, there will be a definite system designed to follow up the issue. This is both a strength and a weakness for the 'consumer'. On the one hand, there are acknowledged pathways through which to complain or seek legal redress; on the other hand, the individual or service that has possibly made a blunder will tend to be protected by the full weight of their institution. People often believe it is pointless to complain because of the strength of the defence mechanisms that protect professionals against external complaints. However, therapists working in the complementary and alternative health fields are not protected by large organisations, but aggrieved 'consumers' could find that the mechanisms through which they can complain are not clear.

6.7   The placebo effect

Orthodox doctors and CAM practitioners view health and healing very differently. Sometimes their views seem very far apart or even irreconcilable. For example, in the late 1990s, the editors of the *New England Journal of Medicine* (one of the world's most prestigious medical journals) declared: 'It is time for the scientific community to stop giving alternative medicine a free ride' (Angell and Kassirer, 1998, p. 841). This attack did not come out of the blue. There has been a long tradition of medical tribalism in which orthodox practitioners attack CAM for being unscientific and CAM practitioners attack orthodoxy for being too mechanistic and disease-focused.

There may be one issue that the two camps can agree about. They are generally comfortable about accepting the existence of a **placebo** effect in most types of treatment, both orthodox and alternative.

What is a placebo and how effective is it?

The placebo effect can be defined in either a narrow or a broad way. The narrow definition refers to the beneficial effects of giving a person a dummy treatment that resembles an active treatment but is biologically inert. For example, a placebo pill might contain only sugar or starch; or the use of a placebo acupuncture needle in a procedure resembling acupuncture but without penetrating the skin (Streitberger and Kleinhenz, 1998).

The broader definition of the placebo effect includes not just the effect of the dummy treatment but also the wide array of non-specific effects in the person–health professional relationship. These include the attention given by the professional, the professional's compassionate care and communication, and the way in which the interaction can modulate the person's expectations, anxiety and self-awareness.

How effective is the placebo effect? One of the first researchers to attempt to answer this question was a physician from Massachusetts General Hospital, Henry Beecher. In his classic study called 'The powerful placebo', published in 1955, Beecher combined the results of 15 different clinical trials in which an active drug was compared with a placebo pill. He found that about one-third of people given a placebo experienced beneficial effects (Beecher, 1955).

Studies done since then give a wide range of figures for the proportion of people who benefit from receiving a placebo. For example, Walsh et al. (2002) looked at 75 placebo-controlled trials of anti-depressant drugs (that is, people were given either an anti-depressant or a placebo) between January 1981 and December 2000. The proportion of people who responded to a placebo ranged from 13 to 52 per cent (the mean was 30 per cent). The proportion was higher in recent trials compared with older trials, although it is unclear why this happened.

Does it matter how often a placebo is given, what colour it is, or whether it is a pill or a device? The following research results suggest that these factors do contribute to a placebo's effectiveness.

- One study found that giving a placebo pill four times a day was more effective than giving it twice a day (de Craen et al., 1999).
- Many studies have compared placebo pills with devices (for example, a starch pill compared with an injection of saline) for treating a wide variety of medical conditions, such as varicose veins and osteoarthritis. These studies found that placebo devices appear to be more effective than placebo pills (Kaptchuk et al., 2000).
- Active placebos, which are specially manufactured to cause side effects (they contain drugs such as atropine to give patients a dry mouth), have a greater effect than inactive placebos (Moncrieff et al., 1998).

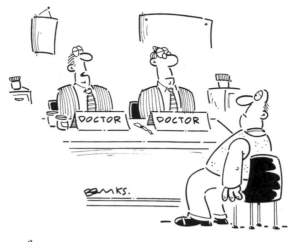

"ONE OF US IS A PLACEBO, MR JONES..."

How does a placebo work?

There are many different theories about how a placebo might work. For example, some researchers argue that what could be considered a placebo effect is merely the body's natural process of healing after an illness or injury, or the natural waxing and waning of any disease process (Di Blasi et al., 2001).

Two particular theories about the beneficial effect of placebos have gained even greater popularity. The first could be called the **psychological** theory (Brody, 2000). This posits that the placebo works because people believe in its healing power. This belief may act through the nervous system to affect the person's hormonal and immune systems. Alternatively, such beliefs may lead people to change their attitude or behaviour, which in turn could have a physical effect on their body.

The second theory could be called the **process of treatment theory**. This theory argues that what matters in the placebo effect is the way in which the health professional shows care and attention to the person who comes for help (Kaptchuk, 2002). This process triggers physical changes in the person that lead to healing. So, it is not the placebo pill itself but the act of a professional giving the pill that matters.

These two theories rely on both the person and the health professional believing in the treatment and this is looked at more closely next.

The importance of people's beliefs

It is unclear why some patients get a beneficial effect from a placebo and others do not. However, one factor seems to be the expectations or beliefs that the person brings to the treatment setting. In a classic experiment in the USA in 1964, people were given a placebo pill and were told, at different times and in random order, that the pill was a bowel relaxant, a bowel stimulant and a dummy pill (Sternbach, 1964). Researchers measured the participants' stomach movements (gastric motility) and found that they were consistent with what the people had been told. Similarly, people with asthma who believed that an inhaler would help them breathe better got symptom relief even when that inhaler was a placebo (Sodergren and Hyland, 1999).

CAM is particularly likely to elicit a powerful placebo response because of the faith that patients may bring to the interaction between client and practitioner. Ted Kaptchuk, of Harvard University's Center for Alternative Medicine Research, argues:

> In contrast to conventional medicine, with its measured objectivity, alternative medicine offers a charged constellation of expectations. Alternative medicine's romantic vision is inhabited by benevolent and intentional forces (for example, the innate intelligence of chiropractic or the *qi* of acupuncture) that are unrestrained by the laws of normative physics. An exaggerated notion of the possible readily elicits patients' magical anticipation.
>
> (Kaptchuk, 2002, p. 818)

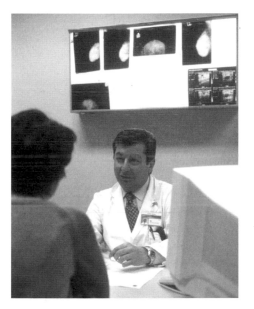

As well as the basic evidence about their illness, people want information based on values that they can understand and relate to: 'Personal experiences I found much more useful than just bland brochures' (Lockwood, 2004, p. 1033)

The importance of professionals' beliefs

In many clinical trials the placebo response is greater when physicians are more optimistic about the treatment than when they are neutral or negative (Uhlenhuth et al., 1966). Similarly, when the same medication is given to people by different physicians there are different responses. For example, one literature review of 25 trials that randomly assigned people with physical illnesses to different levels of expectancy by professionals about the treatment found that: 'enhancing patients' expectations through positive information about the treatment or the illness, while providing support or reassurance, [seemed to] significantly influence health outcomes' (Di Blasi et al., 2001, p. 757).

CAM practitioners tend to be more upbeat and positive than orthodox health professionals about the treatments they offer, which could be an important factor in the enhanced placebo effect seen with CAM.

How should the success of treatment be measured?

Some treatments, particularly CAM treatments, have an enhanced placebo effect. This raises an important philosophical question that gets to the heart of the tensions between CAM and orthodox medicine: 'How should the success of treatment be measured?' In orthodox medicine, a treatment is said to be effective if it works better than a placebo. However, the problem with this approach is that it risks denigrating the placebo effect as being 'bogus' – a treatment can only be 'real' if its effect is greater than this 'bogus' effect.

Now consider a person who goes to a health professional, receives a placebo treatment, and feels healed. Has the treatment been a 'success'? Can it be called real healing if it was 'just a bogus' placebo that led to the improvement?

There are no right or wrong answers to these questions. There are clearly cultural and social judgements about what constitutes 'real' healing. For example, some people believe that if acupuncture helps a person, it was 'only' a placebo effect. Assume for a moment that this is true. Does it matter? The person believes they have benefited, and the mechanism by which they have benefited makes no difference.

In conventional, evidence-based medicine, practitioners attempt to remove the placebo effect when appraising a new treatment, at the risk of 'throwing the baby out with the bath water'. On the other hand, CAM practitioners accept that the placebo effect is part of healing, and do what they can to enhance this effect. Yamey (2000) argues that where evidence-based medicine has let doctors and patients down is in ignoring the non-specific, 'complex effects' that are a crucial part of the healing process. Randomised controlled trials attempt to eliminate factors such as the therapeutic setting, the personality of the therapist, the amount of time given to patients, and even the words spoken to them. Instead of being hidden in the placebo part of the experiment, these factors should be disentangled and studied systematically, so that their therapeutic benefits can be harnessed by everyone involved in providing health care.

6.8   Conclusion

This chapter discussed some aspects of orthodox medical practice. We hope that it showed some of the ways in which certain orthodox medical concerns are similar to those that influence the practice of complementary and alternative health care and that it answered the following questions. Does the intervention work? In what ways can this type of practice claim success? What problems are associated with the use and abuse of these practices?

The focus was on evidence-based medicine (EBM). This has developed into a specific set of indicators that are designed to demonstrate whether particular interventions are effective – or not. The imposition of this set of EBM rules on top of all orthodox medical practice has its problems, which were outlined in this chapter. Even more problems are associated with attempts to use EBM as a tool for assessing complementary and alternative forms of treatment. In addition, EBM does not seem very good at wider considerations, such as whether the introduction of a particular treatment that has been shown to be 'effective' for individuals may have wider effects on the population's health.

The power of many forms of orthodox medicine to do good was also explored. However, it can be difficult to control this power and some of the adverse effects resulting from the practice of orthodox medicine were discussed.

Finally, the placebo effect was scrutinised and some of the ways in which this effect is conceptualised within the orthodox medical sphere were explored.

KEY POINTS

■ When studying complementary and alternative health issues it is also important to think critically about the dominant orthodox medical system.

■ The origins of orthodox medicine can be traced back to very fundamental, scientific roots. The logic of the scientific method continues to inform the way in which orthodox medicine is practised currently.

■ Many important medical advances throughout history have been the result of the application of scientific methodology to the study of human functioning and malfunctioning.

■ Evidence-based medicine has achieved considerable dominance within the medical establishment through the application of rigorous methodology to establish whether particular interventions are beneficial — or not.

■ The use of EBM has its own limitations and some interventions cannot be measured in this way.

■ There are significant problems associated with the use of orthodox medicine in individuals; side effects and other adverse effects can create significant problems.

■ The placebo effect is potentially an important part of every intervention in both orthodox medicine and CAM.

References

Abraham, J. (2002) 'Making regulation responsive to commercial interests: streamlining drug industry watchdogs', *British Medical Journal*, Vol. 325, pp. 1164–9.

Andrews, L. B., Stocking, C., Krizek, T., Gottlieb, I., Krizek, C., Vargish, T. et al. (1997) 'An alternative strategy for studying adverse events in medical care', *The Lancet*, Vol. 349, pp. 309–13.

Angell, M. and Kassirer, J. P. (1998) Editorial: 'Alternative medicine – the risks of untested and unregulated remedies', *The New England Journal of Medicine*, Vol. 339, No. 12, pp. 839–41.

Antman, E., Lau, J., Kupelnick, B., Mosteller, F. and Chalmers, C. (1992) 'A comparison of results of meta-analyses of randomized control trials and recommendations of experts', *Journal of the American Medical Association*, Vol. 268, pp. 240–8.

Audit Commission (2001) *A Spoonful of Sugar*, London, Audit Commission.

Bacon, F. (1605) *The Advancement of Learning. Book I*, London, Henrie Tomes.

Beecher, H. (1955) 'The powerful placebo', *Journal of the American Medical Association*, Vol. 159, No. 17, pp. 1602–6.

Berwick, D. and Leape, L. (1999) 'Reducing errors in medicine', *British Medical Journal*, Vol. 319, pp. 136–7.

Blendon, R., Schoen, C., DesRoches, C., Osborn, R. and Zapert, K. (2003) 'Common concerns amid diverse systems: health care experiences in five countries', *Health Affairs*, Vol. 22, No. 3, pp. 106–21. Available online at: www.healthaffairs.org/readeragent.php?ID=/usr/local/apache/sites/healthaffairs.org/htdocs/Library/v22n3/s17.pdf [accessed 10 June 2003].

Brennan, A., Leape, L., Laird, N., Hebert, L., Localio, R. and Lawthers, A. (1991) 'Incidence of adverse events and negligence in hospitalised patients', *The New England Journal of Medicine*, Vol. 324, pp. 370–84.

British National Formulary (2004) *BNF48* [online], www.bnf.org/ [accessed 19 November 2004].

Brody, H. (2000) 'The placebo response', *The Journal of Family Practice*, Vol. 49, No. 7, pp. 649–54.

Choudhury, N., Stelfox, H. and Detsky, A. (2002) 'Relationships between authors of clinical practice guidelines and the pharmaceutical industry', *Journal of the American Medical Association*, Vol. 287, No. 5, pp. 612–7.

Cochrane Collaboration (2004) Website: www.cochrane.org/index0.htm [accessed 19 November 2004].

de Craen, A. J., Moerman, D. E., Heisterkamp, S. H., Tytgat, G. N., Tijssen, J. G. and Kleijnen, J. (1999) 'Placebo effect in the treatment of duodenal ulcer', *British Journal of Clinical Pharmacology*, Vol. 48, pp. 853–60.

Di Blasi, Z., Harkness, E., Ernst, E., Georgiou, A. and Kleijnen, J. (2001) 'Influence of context effects on health outcomes: a systematic review', *The Lancet*, Vol. 357, pp. 757–62.

Donald, A. (2002) 'Evidence-based medicine: key concepts', *Medscape General Medicine*, Vol. 4, No. 2 [online], www.medscape.com/viewarticle/430709 [accessed 4 February 2005].

Donchin, Y., Gopher, D., Olin, M., Badihi, Y., Biesky, M., Sprung, C. L. et al. (1995) 'A look into the nature and causes of human errors in the intensive care unit', *Critical Care Medicine*, Vol. 23, pp. 294–300.

Doorey, A., Michelson, E. and Topol, E. (1992) 'Thrombolytic therapy of acute myocardial infarction', *Journal of the American Medical Association*, Vol. 268, pp. 3108–14.

Ebrahim, S. (1999) 'Systematic review of cost-effectiveness research of stroke evaluation and treatment', *Stroke*, Vol. 30, No. 12, pp. 2759–60.

Freeman, A. C. and Sweeney, K. (2001) 'Why general practitioners do not implement evidence: qualitative study', *British Medical Journal*, Vol. 323, pp. 1100–2.

Harvey, W. (1628) *An Anatomical Study of the Motion of the Heart and of the Blood in Animals*, Frankfurt, W. Fitzer.

Haynes, R. (2002) 'What kind of evidence is it that evidence-based medicine advocates want health care providers and consumers to pay attention to?', *British Medical Council Health Services Research*, Vol. 2, No. 1, p. 3.

Heller, R. and Dobson, A. (2000) 'Disease impact number and population impact number: a population perspective to measures of risk and benefit', *British Medical Journal*, Vol. 321, pp. 950–2.

Heller, R. and Page, J. (2002) 'A population perspective to evidence based medicine: "evidence for population health"', *Journal of Epidemiology and Community Health*, Vol. 56, pp. 45–7.

Hitt, J. (2001) 'Evidence-based medicine, *New York Times Magazine*, 9 December, Section 6, pp. 68–69.

Illich, I. (1976) *Limits to Medicine*, London, Marion Boyars.

Kaptchuk, T. J. (2002) 'The placebo effect in alternative medicine: can the performance of a healing ritual have clinical significance?', *Annals of Internal Medicine*, Vol. 136, pp. 817–25.

Kaptchuk, T., Goldman, P., Stone, D. and Stason, W. (2000) 'Do medical devices have enhanced placebo effects?', *Journal of Clinical Epidemiology*, Vol. 53, pp. 786–92.

Ketley, D. and Woods, K. (1993) 'Impact of clinical trials on clinical practice: example of thrombolysis for acute myocardial infarction', *The Lancet*, Vol. 342, pp. 891–4.

Koch, R. (1882) 'Mycobacterium tuberculosis', Lecture to Physiological Society of Berlin, 24 March.

Leibovici, L. and Lièvre, M. (2002) Editorial – 'Medicalisation: peering from inside medicine', *British Medical Journal*, Vol. 324, p. 866.

Lexchin, J., Bero, L., Djulbegovic, B. and Clark, O. (2003) 'Pharmaceutical industry sponsorship and research outcome and quality: systematic review', *British Medical Journal*, Vol. 326, pp. 1167–70.

Lockwood, S. (2004) '"Evidence of me" in evidence-based medicine?', *British Medical Journal*, Vol. 329, pp. 1033–35.

Mair, F., Crowley, T. and Bundred, P. (1996) 'Prevalence, aetiology and management of heart failure in general practice', *British Journal of General Practice*, Vol. 46, pp. 77–9.

Mashru, M. and Lant, A. (1997) 'Interpractice audit of diagnosis and management of hypertension in primary care: educational intervention and review of medical records', *British Medical Journal*, Vol. 314, pp. 942–6.

Medical Research Council Streptomycin in Tuberculosis Trials Committee (1948) 'Streptomycin treatment for pulmonary tuberculosis', *British Medical Journal*, Vol. 2, pp. 769–82.

Moncrieff, J., Wessely, S. and Hardy, R. (1998) 'Meta-analysis of trials comparing antidepressants with active placebos', *British Journal of Psychiatry*, Vol. 172, pp. 227–31.

Moynihan, R. (2003) 'Who pays for the pizza? Redefining the relationship between doctors and drug companies', *British Medical Journal*, Vol. 326, pp. 1189–92 and 1193–6.

Prosser, H., Almond, S. and Walley, T. (2003) 'Influences on GPs' decision to prescribe new drugs – the importance of who says what', *Family Practice*, Vol. 20, No. 1, pp. 61–8.

Sackett, D., Rosenberg, W., Gray, J., Haynes, R. and Richardson, W. (1996) Editorial – 'Evidence based medicine: what it is and what it isn't', *British Medical Journal*, Vol. 312, pp. 71–2.

Sodergren, S. and Hyland, M. (1999) 'Expectancy and asthma', in Kirsch, I. (ed.) *How Expectancies Shape Experience*, Washington, DC, American Psychological Association.

Sternbach, R. (1964) 'The effects of instructional sets on autonomic responsivity', *Psychophysiology*, Vol. 62, pp. 67–72.

Streitberger, K. and Kleinhenz, J. (1998) 'Introducing a placebo needle into acupuncture research', *The Lancet*, Vol. 352, pp. 364–5.

Sudlow, M., Rodgers, H., Kenny, R. and Thomson, R. (1997) 'Population based study of use of anticoagulants among patients with a trial fibrillation in the community', *British Medical Journal*, Vol. 314, pp. 1529–30.

Uhlenhuth, E., Rickels, K., Fisher, S., Park, L., Lipman, R. and Mock, J. (1966) 'Drug, doctors' verbal attitude and clinic setting in the symptomatic response to pharmacotherapy', *Psychopharmacologia*, Vol. 9, pp. 392–418.

Vincent, C., Neale, G. and Woloshynowych, M. (2001) 'Adverse events in British hospitals: preliminary retrospective record review', *British Medical Journal*, Vol. 322, pp. 517–9.

Walsh, B. T., Seidman, S. N., Sysko, R. and Gould, M. (2002) 'Placebo response in studies of major depression: variable, substantial, and growing', *Journal of the American Medical Association*, Vol. 287, pp. 1840–7.

Weingart, S. N., Wilson, R. M., Gibberd, R. W. and Harrison, B. (2000) 'Epidemiology of medical error', *British Medical Journal*, Vol. 320, pp. 774–7.

Wilson, R., Runciman, W., Gibberd, R., Harrison, B., Newby, L. and Hamilton, J. (1995) 'The quality in Australian health care study', *Medical Journal of Australia*, Vol. 163, pp. 458–71.

World Health Organization (2003) *WHO Policy and Strategy on Traditional Medicine*, Geneva, World Health Organization. Available online at: www.who.int/medicines/organization/trm/orgtrmmain.shtml [accessed 8 August 2003].

Yamey, G. (2000) 'Can complementary medicine be evidence based?', *Western Journal of Medicine*, Vol. 173, pp. 4–5.

Chapter 7 Understanding research

Hilary MacQueen, Sheena Murdoch and Andrew Vickers

Contents

AIMS

- To examine the meaning of 'research'.
- To describe the standards and techniques used in biomedical research.
- To explore the debate about whether biomedical research standards and techniques are appropriate for researching CAM.

7.1 Introduction

A recurring theme in this book so far is the need to establish a research base for complementary and alternative medicine (CAM). This was evident when countering accusations of fraud, vital in providing appropriate education and training for CAM practitioners and fundamental in gaining professional status and statutory self-regulation. This raises the thorny issue of what type of research is applicable to CAM. In Chapter 6 the close relationship between orthodox medicine and the scientific method was discussed. This chapter focuses on health research and its application to CAM. It begins by asking what is research, how is it done, and why do it? It goes on to consider the variety of methodologies available to researchers, showing how some are readily applicable to CAM research. Finally, the present and future roles of CAM research are examined.

7.2 What is research?

Research is about methodical investigation, discovery and explanation, to collect information or to establish facts and principles that will add to the body of knowledge about a phenomenon. There are contested theories about what 'knowledge' is. The study of these theories is called **epistemology**, which concerns what is or should be considered acceptable, legitimate and valid knowledge and the methods used to obtain it.

Epistemological questions about the validity of knowledge and the methods used to obtain it rest on questions about the form and nature of phenomena, such as what is the form and nature of reality or what is the form and nature of existence? Different views about the form and nature of phenomena or entities are frequently referred to as 'world views', 'paradigms' or ontological 'positions' or 'perspectives'. The latter term is often used because 'ontology' is the branch of philosophy concerning the nature of existence and so questions about the form and nature of phenomena are considered to be questions of ontology.

World views, what constitutes valid and legitimate knowledge and the methods used to obtain that knowledge are interlinked. In the fields of orthodox medicine and CAM debate continues about two different world views and whether they can be investigated in the same manner. These world views are often called 'reductionism' and 'holism'. **Reductionism** is the practice of reducing observable phenomena or biological processes to their constituent parts in order to analyse them and the relationships between them. A reductionist world view usually emphasises objective measures and quantitative (statistical) methods of research. Orthodox medicine (or biomedicine) is frequently associated with a reductionist world view. **Holism** is a view of health in which the physical, social and spiritual aspects of a person are considered to be inseparable. Many CAM therapies are characterised by their holistic approach to health. Questions arise from this holistic approach about whether research on CAM requires different methods from those conventionally used for researching orthodox medicine. The answers to these questions are underpinned by what each world view will accept as valid and legitimate knowledge and evidence.

There is another debate running parallel to this debate. In the expanding, complex and diverse arena of health many new research questions are being asked. Debate is ongoing about whether the research methods conventionally used in much biomedical research are adequate for exploring all types of research questions that arise in health and health services provision.

The next section looks in detail at 'the scientific method'. This is one theory of what constitutes valid knowledge and how to obtain it. The logic of this method is often thought to underpin biomedicine. It is associated with the reductionist world view that is currently the most dominant influence on health care research in western society. You will probably encounter this approach when reading about and using research on both orthodox medicine and CAM. People in authority often regard the principles that underpin biomedicine and biomedicine's definition of what constitutes evidence as more accurate and credible than other perspectives on what constitutes valid knowledge. However, much of the debate about how to research CAM arose from concern about whether and to what extent the research standards and techniques used in biomedical research are appropriate for researching CAM.

7.3   The biomedical perspective and scientific research

Many diverse claims have been made about health. Some of them appear to be comparatively uncontroversial: for example, the use of antibiotics is good for severe bacterial infections. Some are currently open to debate: such as the possible link between pesticides and cancer. Many others, such as the value of bloodletting or severe purges for fever, have now been discarded in most cultures.

ACTIVITY   HEALTH CLAIMS

Allow 10 minutes

Box 7.1 lists a wide variety of health claims made by biomedical scientists, CAM practitioners, businesses, advocacy groups and members of the lay public. Try to identify which group made each claim.

BOX 7.1   EXAMPLES OF HEALTH CLAIMS

1   Antibiotics are of value for severe bacterial infections
2   Pesticides cause cancer
3   Flora® reduces the risk of heart disease
4   Acupuncture can help back pain
5   Vaccination causes autism
6   Sepsis from *Pneumococcus aeruginosa* induces a p53-independent decrease in gut epithelial proliferation
7   Masturbation retards intellectual and emotional development
8   It is safe to take thalidomide in pregnancy
9   Genetically modified foods are safe to eat
10 Geranium oil is effective for diabetes
11 Chicken soup is good for the common cold
12 Red foods are bad for arthritis
13 A baby who kicks in the womb will be a boy
14 Bleeding is a good treatment for fever
15 Women's wombs make them prone to nervous diseases
16 Babies should be born in hospital

Comment

You probably did not have too much trouble identifying who made these claims. The key question is have all claims been in the best interests of users and public health in general? The answer, of course, is no. It is widely accepted that many historical medical practices were misplaced or even barbaric and that some claims made by advocacy groups and businesses are very questionable.

How can the validity of health claims be assessed? How are views and beliefs about the best way to tackle health issues established? And why are some views that were passionately held in particular cultures at certain times later discarded in favour of other, equally passionately held views? Research has an important function in establishing, enhancing or invalidating the credibility of different approaches, practices and treatments. One way of thinking about research is to see it as a set of procedures designed to help determine the value of different views and beliefs.

Exactly how should the credibility of a practice or treatment be established or invalidated? What is regarded as acceptable, warranted evidence or knowledge on which to base decisions about health care? Current clinical and biomedical perspectives about what constitutes valid research and evidence are usually based on the principles of the **scientific method**. Before looking at these principles in general, the purpose of research is explored by focusing on clinical trials, a way in which biomedicine attempts to assess the value of claims about treatment.

The purpose of clinical trials

When a new treatment is devised to address a particular health condition, two questions need to be asked: 'Does the treatment work?' and 'Is it safe to use?' These questions cannot be answered satisfactorily without thorough research. When Frederick Banting and Charles Best discovered in the early 1920s that one form of diabetes mellitus results from a lack of the pancreatic hormone insulin, the logical deduction was that diabetes could be treated by giving insulin to the affected person (Banting, 1925). However, theory had to be borne out by practice, and it had to be shown whether insulin that was not made in a diabetic person's body would still work in this environment and without causing harm. The dose, the frequency and the route of delivery (for example, orally, topically or by injection) also had to be determined. In Banting and Best's day, these areas were investigated in a rather ad hoc manner (see Box 7.2). This lack of standard, thorough investigative practice led to some horrific medical accidents, such as the thalidomide tragedy in the late 1950s and early 1960s.

BOX 7.2   BANTING, BEST AND MARJORIE, THE DIABETIC DOG

Diabetes is a disease in which people cannot metabolise their food properly, particularly sugar. If left untreated, many diabetic people waste away and die a few months after the onset of the disease. In the early 20th century, hospital wards were full of 'living skeletons' — diabetic people waiting to die. The source of the problem for some of them was known to be a set of cells called the islets of Langerhans after their discoverer, the German pathologist Paul Langerhans (1847—1888). These cells are located in the pancreas, a gland that lies behind the stomach. However, it was not known what the problem within the pancreas actually was.

In 1920, the Canadian doctor Frederick Banting had returned from service in the First World War and was struggling to make ends meet. He took a teaching job at Western University in London, Ontario. While writing notes for a lecture on the pancreas, he had an idea for an experiment. He planned to remove the pancreas from a dog, making it diabetic, then to make extracts of the removed pancreas and try to restore health by giving the extracts back to the dog. He was helped in this endeavour by a student, Charles Best. Banting performed the surgery and Best measured sugar levels in the dog's blood and urine. After a few false starts, they got their experiment to work, and their laboratory dog, Marjorie, was kept alive by injections of pancreatic extract for 70 days after her pancreas was removed.

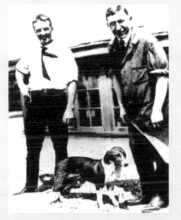

Frederick Banting (right) and Charles Best

Eventually, in 1921, the extract was purified down to a single active substance, which was called **insulin**, from the Latin word *insula* meaning 'island'. The discovery of a treatment for diabetes made Banting and Best heroes, and Banting became Canada's first Nobel laureate, in 1923. Sadly, Best was not credited; instead, the head of the laboratory, J. J. R. MacLeod, shared the prize. Banting gave half of his to Best, and continued to work on insulin. He was knighted in 1934.

Insulin is not a cure for diabetes, only a treatment for some forms of the disease. Currently in Canada, diabetes and its complications is still a leading cause of death.

The level of regulation of the pharmaceutical industry is very high, partly because of frustration at the lack of a 'gold standard' (a test against which all others are measured) in drug testing, and partly because of legislation arising from people's concern about issues such as thalidomide. In the Medicines Act 1968, the most recent legislation stipulates a protocol of testing for efficacy and safety for any new treatment. Such treatments generally involve new chemicals, but the legislation covers the use of devices and procedures too, although, interestingly, many herbal remedies are exempt from the terms of the Act. However, its major application is in the development of new chemicals – drugs. The choice of chemical to be synthesised is based on a good understanding of the science of the biological system and the condition affecting it. Many different chemicals are made and screened (tested) to see whether they have any effect that might prove beneficial. The screening is done *in vitro* (that is, on isolated chemicals, cells and tissues, not on whole animals or humans) by automated, robotic processes in a laboratory.

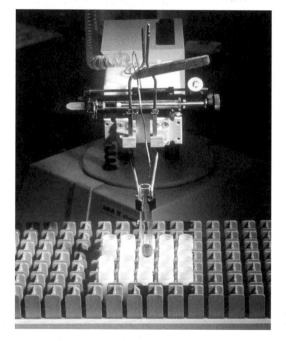

An automated system for handling test samples

Once a chemical is identified as promising, it has to be tested using the following protocol.

- **Initial production**: enough of the chemical needs to be produced for all the testing.
- **Pre-clinical trials**: carried out mainly on animals. This is pharmacological testing to establish what the drug does, how it acts, in what form it is best administered, how long it stays active in the body, and the route by

which it is eliminated. It also involves toxicity testing to establish how poisonous it is (remember that there is no such thing as a completely safe drug). This is the longest and most expensive phase of drug testing.

■ **Phase I clinical trials**: the first contact humans have with the drug. Small numbers of volunteers are tested in planned, controlled experiments lasting up to a year. This is the point at which the toxicity and the pharmacological data obtained in pre-clinical trials are checked for their validity in humans.

■ **Phase II clinical trials**: the large-scale testing of the drug. This stage may last up to two years and involves several hundred volunteers, some of whom have the condition which the drug is designed to address. This is the stage at which double-blind, placebo-controlled randomised trials or RCTs (described later in this section) are carried out. This is the 'acid test' for whether the drug really is effective. It can also establish the optimum dosage.

■ **Phase III clinical trials**: the evaluation, by comparative studies, of the best regime for administering the drug, either alone or in combination with another substance, intermittently or continuously, etc. This stage involves large numbers of people with the disease or condition and lasts three years or more. Because so many people are involved in the trials, even rare side effects are likely to be picked up. However, some adverse effects may go unnoticed, and there must be constant post-marketing monitoring of side effects. This is currently achieved by a 'yellow card' system, in which practitioners report symptoms experienced by their patients to a central database, where reports are collated. Any emerging risks can then be publicised.

A certificate approving the drug can be obtained only when there have been satisfactory results in the trials and only then can a product licence application be made.

The entire process from drug synthesis to marketing can take 10 years and cost hundreds of millions of pounds, which goes some way to explain the high costs involved in drug development. There is only a 0.01 per cent chance of a drug identified by screening as potentially useful reaching the market and making money for the company (Kettler, 2001). This means pharmaceutical companies, and the people working for them, are under great pressure to 'deliver' a blockbuster drug, which is active against a common complaint and will give good financial returns for the shareholders. The patent life of a new compound is 15 years, so if it takes 10 years from discovery to market, there are only five years of patent protection left before so-called generic drugs (chemically similar compounds that act on the body in a very similar way) can be sold, generally more cheaply than the parent compound. Note that CAM remedies cannot be patented because they are natural products.

So, many pharmaceutical companies concentrate on drugs that they can sell in the rich, developed world for financial reasons. They are less willing to develop drugs that are unlikely to make money because the conditions that they treat are either rare or common only in poor countries with small health budgets. As clinical trials progress, expenditure escalates and it becomes increasingly important to the company that the drug eventually makes a good profit. Drug development and marketing are very expensive processes, and only large companies have the resources to underwrite them.

Faced with the huge amounts of money involved in fulfilling legal requirements for efficacy and safety testing, how can notoriously under-funded CAM compete? The short answer is that it can't. Unless there is a compelling reason to investigate a particular CAM remedy so that funding can be made available, it simply will not be done. In many cases the best that can be hoped for is that some form of trial, probably on a fairly small scale, can be carried out, and that the subsequent data analysis will yield significant results. Sceptics frequently cite the paucity of significant data as a reason for not using CAM, but a body of evidence is gradually emerging from smaller, cheaper trials that allows some CAM remedies to be considered on equal terms with costly pharmaceuticals.

The scientific method

As described above, pharmaceutical products have to go through lengthy and expensive testing protocols, but this chapter has not yet addressed the question of **why** such long-winded assessments are necessary. Why is it simply not good enough for a practitioner to say, 'Well, I've used treatment X on hundreds of people, and it usually works' and for the wider community to accept that treatment X is valid? The reasons boil down to what is acceptable as a true and fair test. To understand this requires a brief journey around the philosophy of science and its operating standard – the scientific method.

According to the philosopher of science Karl Popper (1902–1994), the most important part of scientific reasoning is the formulation of a **hypothesis** (Popper, 1959). This is a provisional explanation of observed phenomena, or even of completely theoretical events. For any system (set of circumstances) there may be many, competing hypotheses, not all of which can be correct. However, a hypothesis allows predictions to be made about how the system will react if its parameters are changed. For example, based on the observation that it never seems to rain when I have my umbrella with me, a hypothesis might be: 'If I take an umbrella out with me today, it will not rain because the umbrella will ward off rain clouds.' A prediction of this hypothesis might then be that if I take an umbrella with me and it is **already** raining (that is, the experimental conditions have changed), the umbrella will ward off clouds and the rain will immediately stop. This prediction can easily be tested by taking an umbrella out in all kinds of weather. It will be shown not to stand up to testing. This example illustrates two important points: the hypothesis must be **testable** by experiment and it must be **falsifiable**, that is, able to be disproved. Crucially, a hypothesis can never be **proved**, as it is impossible to say that a hypothesis is correct in all circumstances – merely that conditions have not yet been devised in which the prediction of the hypothesis has failed to occur. The results of the tests can only be said to be **consistent with** the hypothesis. The whole purpose of scientific research is therefore to formulate hypotheses based on observations or theoretical predictions, and then to test the hypotheses as thoroughly as possible, **with the aim of disproving them**. The latter phrase is emphasised because scientists are only human. If there is a large body of evidence supporting a favourite hypothesis, the motivation to continue testing the hypothesis may flag somewhat!

ACTIVITY   FORMULATING A HYPOTHESIS

Allow 5 minutes

Try to formulate the hypothesis tested by Banting and Best in their study of diabetes mellitus (described in Box 7.2).

Comment

The hypothesis was that a substance made by the pancreas can restore health in diabetic dogs.

The testing of a hypothesis follows a clearly defined set of steps called the **scientific method** of research. The aim is to give the scientist a defence against allegations of vested interest by trying to disprove the hypothesis. Of course, it is vital to maintain objectivity in observing and interpreting test results, which implies including appropriate controls in experiments (that is, sets of experimental conditions in which the outcomes can be predicted with certainty, and taken as baseline values against which to make comparisons). Experiments are done in a systematic way – that is, by an agreed sequence of steps – so that any scientist should be able to replicate another's findings. Replication and reproducibility are vital to demonstrate the credibility of research. The end-point of the test (that is, what is measured and when) must be clearly stated: for example, are results collected after a particular time, or when a desired outcome is achieved, whenever that may be? Results must be peer-reviewed before they are accepted, and this system of the application of standard protocols and internal policing, while not completely foolproof, is widely accepted as yielding robust and reproducible data. The data may be consistent with the hypothesis being tested, so that the hypothesis remains a viable possibility, or they may not, in which case the hypothesis can be rejected, and an alternative formulated that takes account of all the existing data, to be tested in its turn.

The description above may help to explain why progress in science often seems painfully slow. While a series of experiments can yield interesting data that may support a new hypothesis, no credible scientist would claim the hypothesis as the answer to life, the universe and everything on the basis of only a few tests. This is a source of friction between scientists and members of the media who are apt to want to trumpet 'latest research' stories, while scientists usually prefer to be more cautious until there is a strong body of incontrovertible data (although obviously there are exceptions). This explains why so many scientists are sceptical about CAM: they may be open-minded but, until there are sufficient data to support the hypothesis that 'treatment X is beneficial for depression', for example, their training and general approach to life simply do not allow them to accept it. (It is worth emphasising here that 'data' can include observation as well as numerical information.) Claims based solely on the personal experiences of one or a few people are not legitimate in this culture.

However, personal experience is valuable for matters of personal preference. For example, although research may highlight the value of exercise, it cannot tell an individual which type of exercise they find easiest and most enjoyable. Personal experience is also essential for interactions between practitioners and clients: empathy, compassion and listening skills cannot readily be derived from reading research papers. The advantage of research is that it is a more reliable basis for understanding health.

This point can be illustrated further by examining some of the problems associated with using personal experience to reach conclusions about health. Consider the following two statements: the first could be from a passionate but uncritical advocate of aromatherapy; the second might have been made by an old-fashioned, ultra-conservative general practitioner (GP).

1   Rose oil is a good treatment for all people with bulimia.
2   All patients who use CAM are neurotic, middle-aged, middle-class women who don't have anything particularly wrong with them.

There are several interesting features about these statements.

■   They are presented as facts, in the same way as a geographer might state that London is south of Glasgow.
■   There is no reference to why the statements are thought to be true: for instance, by using phrases such as 'recent research has demonstrated' or 'in the clinical experience of aromatherapists' or even 'it seems reasonable to suppose'.

■ The statements are general: they are not about a particular person or even group of people. In addition, they are intended to be applied: that is, everyone with bulimia should consider rose oil; any doctor who has a consultation with someone using CAM should realise they are not sick in any way.

When challenged to defend their statements, both the aromatherapist and the GP might claim that they were based on personal experience. Is individual experience a valid basis for making universal generalisations? From the perspective of the scientific method, there are several problems associated with personal experience.

Observation

Observation, as described above, is often the basis of designing a hypothesis, but what people observe is often influenced by what they believe. A good example is an optical illusion in which what is seen depends on innate beliefs about shapes, perspective and so on. People's prejudices and values can affect both what they perceive and what they look for. It is not hard to imagine that a person might report an improvement in bulimia because they want to believe that the treatment worked. Similarly, a GP's assessment of a client's health might be influenced by knowledge of whether they used CAM.

A related problem is that a practitioner's main source of information about the effects of their treatment is often self-reporting by the user: for example, a person with bulimia is treated with rose oil and tells the aromatherapist they are doing better; the aromatherapist then believes that the rose oil helped. The problem is that several psychological issues can

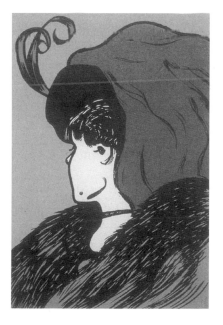

What people see is often influenced by what they want to see. For example, in this optical illusion some people will see a young woman and others will see an older woman. It is not possible to see them both at the same time. Could practitioners' evaluations of the people who consult them be affected by their values and beliefs?

influence what a client tells a practitioner. For example, some people might be embarrassed to say that they are no better, or they may exaggerate their progress to encourage the practitioner. Alternatively, they may report less improvement than they truly experienced, simply because they have forgotten how bad they were. Similarly, a sick person may not tell their GP they are using CAM, especially if they fear a negative response. The GP could then assume that any improvement was a result of the conventional treatment given.

Sampling

Sampling is the selection of particular individuals or results as being representative of all individuals or results. It is an area fraught with hazards. Everybody tends to remember their successes, or instances that illustrate their beliefs particularly well, but the cases that stick in their minds may not represent the true story. If a practitioner sees 10 people who have a particular disease, three may not complete the treatment, five may improve a little and two may improve a great deal. The practitioner will tend to remember the two successful examples and use them as the basis for writing and teaching. Similarly, the hypothetical GP quoted above may tend to remember one or two particularly difficult people who used CAM, and forget the many others who use it without problems or without their GP's knowledge.

There is a further issue concerning the total number of people a practitioner can use as a basis for personal experience. For example, how many people with bulimia does the average aromatherapist see? Are they likely to form a good cross-section of all people with bulimia, or just, say, upper-middle-class women? Similarly, are the doctor's 'worried well' patients representative of all CAM users, or just those in a particular local area or at a certain stage of their illness?

Co-interventions

People tend not to use therapies in isolation: in particular, most people who consult a CAM therapist use conventional medicine concurrently. In this situation the different treatments are known as **co-interventions** and make it almost impossible to tell which therapy helped what condition. For example, in the bulimia case a person could also seek psychotherapy and practise meditation. Yet if that client gets better, the aromatherapist may conclude that the rose oil had helped.

Non-specific factors in healing

A person visiting an aromatherapist receives time and attention as well as a particular aromatherapy oil. They are also likely to have a massage and to spend time in a pleasant and supportive therapeutic environment. Factors such as attention or touch are described as 'non-specific' because they are common to many therapies and contrast with the 'specific' characteristics of a particular therapy, such as an essential oil in aromatherapy or a manipulation in chiropractic. One of the most important non-specific factors is the person's belief that treatment will be beneficial, which is sometimes called the **placebo effect** (see Chapter 6 and the discussion below). Practitioners tend to ascribe a person's improvement to specific aspects of treatment such as the administration of rose oil, rather than to non-specific factors such as care and attention. However, it is generally very difficult to know for certain which aspect worked.

Natural course of disease

Many episodes of illness are self-healing, and people often get better without treatment. (Remember that self-healing processes are precisely those which CAM interventions aim to tap into.) In the case of chronic disease, people have times when they feel better and other times when they feel worse. As they tend to visit practitioners when they are not doing well, they might be expected to start feeling better irrespective of any treatment. A particularly interesting consideration is that people often consult practitioners not when their symptoms peak but just before this happens. Accordingly, they might get worse before they get better, a phenomenon that practitioners may describe as a 'therapeutic crisis' (see Figure 7.1 overleaf).

The idea that the natural course of a disease may compromise opinions based on personal experience is of particular interest when considering **causes** of disease. For example, some parents have claimed that their children became autistic after a vaccination and have joined campaigns against vaccination on the grounds that it causes autism (Leask and McIntyre, 2003). Similarly, there have been cases where a child develops leukaemia shortly after moving to a house near overhead power lines and the parents have concluded that these caused the leukaemia (Czyz et al., 2004). Of course, these children might have developed autism or leukaemia regardless of the vaccination or the house move.

Concordance

Using the term 'compliance' to describe how closely a person follows a practitioner's directives is value-laden and evokes issues of power, belief and trust. It is rather outdated (although still widely used) and the preferred term now is **concordance**. In practice, concordance is a rather thorny issue, as shown by the following example. An aromatherapist gives rose oil to two people who have bulimia. One uses it every day in baths and oil burners; the other does not use the oil at all. Only the person who uses the rose oil gets better.

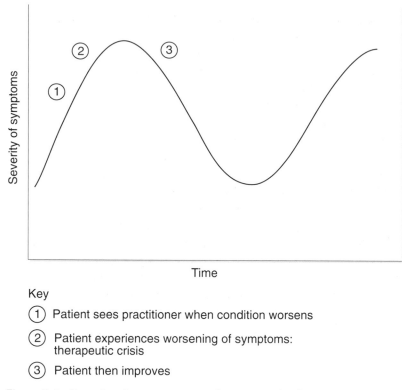

Key

① Patient sees practitioner when condition worsens

② Patient experiences worsening of symptoms: therapeutic crisis

③ Patient then improves

Figure 7.1   Severity of symptoms over the course of a disease

It is tempting to see this as evidence that rose oil is effective. However, there are several other explanations for the apparent link between the use of rose oil and recovery. People who are concordant and follow a practitioner's instructions are also more likely to look after themselves in other ways.
In one famous study, patients who took a sugar pill regularly did better than those who took their sugar pill infrequently (Sackett et al., 1996). This was not because the sugar pill itself was effective but because the people who took it regularly probably paid more attention to themselves, their feelings and their environment, so they remembered to take the pill regularly.

How to avoid errors in research systematically

One of the first lessons people learn in a science practical class is to wash the equipment carefully before using it. If they are trying to see what happens when two chemicals are mixed, it is no good if another chemical is left in the test tube from the previous experiment. Students are also taught to double-check everything. For example, two people working on an experiment together might confirm each step as follows: 'We need to add the acid to the alcohol'; 'That's right: here are the two bottles'; 'Okay, yes, this is the acid and this is the alcohol. I will put both of them in this beaker'; 'Yes, that's right, go on'. Cleaning scientific equipment and double-checking are examples of **systematic attempts to avoid error**. Over the years, researchers have made mistakes and tried to work out where they went wrong. They then incorporate techniques to help avoid making these mistakes again.

Consider the example of the two health beliefs stated earlier about the use of rose oil to treat bulimia and the socioeconomic characteristics of CAM users. These statements can be formulated as hypotheses. Different research methods could be used to test each hypothesis: a clinical trial and a population-based survey respectively. Clinical trials are probably the most well known type of medical research. In a typical trial, participants receive either a treatment or a **placebo**, that is, a treatment without any value that is designed to mimic the real therapy. In the Phase II trial of a drug, for example, participants may take a pill that looks, tastes and smells like the real drug but does not contain any of the drug's active ingredients. Some subjects may have no intervention at all. Who gets the real treatment, no treatment or a placebo is decided **at random** in a similar way to flipping a coin (although the allocation is now often done by a computer). Importantly, neither the subject, the doctor nor anyone else involved in the trial knows who received which treatment. In technical terms, they are **blind** to the treatment allocation. Accordingly, such a trial is known as a **randomised, double-blind, placebo-controlled trial** or sometimes just **double-blind trial** for short. At the end of the trial, the results in the treatment group and the placebo group (and, if appropriate, the no treatment group) are compared to see who did better.

A double-blind trial helps avoid the problems associated with using personal experience in the following ways.

- **Observation**: neither participants nor their practitioners know whether they received the treatment and so will not be influenced to give a better or a worse assessment.
- **Sampling**: in clinical trials, data from all subjects are recorded, not just from those who respond well.
- **Co-interventions**: there are at least two groups of participants and, because they are selected at random, the use of other treatments could be expected to be similar in each group. However, note that this assumption is questionable and any co-interventions should also be recorded.
- **Non-specific factors**: both groups of subjects receive care and attention and a treatment that they believe could help them.
- **Natural course of disease**: comparing the treatment group with the placebo or no treatment control group helps determine whether people would have improved on their own, without any therapy.
- **Concordance**: comparing all the people in both (or all) groups avoids linking concordance with improvement.

Researchers might conduct a population-based survey to determine the characteristics of CAM users. They send a questionnaire to a group of people who are randomly selected from the population as a whole. The questions might be about demographic factors (such as age and gender), medical history and recent use of CAM therapies. The questionnaires are returned anonymously and the results are tabulated. The characteristics of people who used CAM can then be compared with the characteristics of those who did not.

Again, a good questionnaire study can avoid problems associated with personal experience in the following ways.

- **Observation**: questionnaires are carefully written, pre-tested and returned anonymously.
- **Sampling**: the responses of all survey participants are analysed, not just those who give interesting responses. In addition, a large random sample is taken to ensure that those taking part in the survey are similar to the population at large.
- **Co-interventions, non-specific factors and the natural course of disease**: these are not relevant to survey research.
- **Concordance**: responses are analysed from all participants, not just those who follow advice about CAM.

Randomised controlled trials

The question most commonly asked about CAM, and possibly the most important question about any treatment, is 'Does it work?' Researchers usually phrase this as 'Does the treatment do more good than harm?' (Silverman and Chalmers, 2001), although it is not straightforward to answer this question because outcome measures of 'good' and 'harm' are different. Both good and harm can be thought of in many different ways. For example, a treatment such as reflexology is unlikely to harm a recipient directly. However, there is a financial cost involved and, if reflexology is ineffective, time and money spent on it might better be spent having another, more effective treatment. The main way of deciding whether a treatment does more good than harm is to conduct a randomised controlled trial or RCT (Silverman and Chalmers, 2001). As described above, in a typical RCT, participants receive one of two treatments. Who receives which is determined at random, but in RCTs it is not essential (or often even possible) for the trials to be double-blind. At the end of the study, the results from patients in each group are compared. RCTs sometimes compare more than two treatments, or one treatment with a control such as a placebo, as in a placebo-controlled trial (discussed above). However, if a treatment for a condition already exists, it must be made available to some of the participants for ethical reasons (World Medical Association, 2000), so the trial is comparing a potential new treatment with an existing one, and with any controls that the researchers want to include.

ACTIVITY   THE VALIDITY OF CLINICAL TRIALS

Allow 20 minutes

One of the best ways of thinking about the value of RCTs is to consider what can go wrong if they are not used. Imagine that a group of surgeons develop a new technique for treating back pain. They are enthusiastic about their technique and decide to conduct a clinical trial. They treat a number of people for 12 months and report that 60 per cent of them had a good outcome. They compare these results with those from a neighbouring hospital, where only about 50 per cent of the people treated are said to have responded to surgery. The surgeons write up a scientific paper which concludes that the new surgical technique 'is effective and improves the outcome in back pain patients.'

Using the information in this section, consider why the surgeons' conclusion might be unsound.

Comment

Problem 1: the surgeons claim that 60 per cent of their patients improved but which 'patients' are included in this calculation? Did they include all the people with back pain or only those with a certain type of pain? Were people who required additional surgical procedures excluded? What about people who had surgical complications or who did not return to the hospital for follow-up? The surgeons may have only included people with a certain type of back pain that has a good prognosis, or they may have excluded those who experienced medical complications after their surgery. This would tend to inflate the apparent effects of treatment.

Solution: a key aspect of an RCT is careful follow-up of all the participants. Researchers set specific inclusion and exclusion criteria for determining who is eligible for the study. They then attempt to obtain data for all the included subjects.

Problem 2: the surgeons compare their results with those of a neighbouring hospital. However, there may be differences among the people attending each hospital other than the type of surgery they received. For example, those in the neighbouring hospital may be older, or poorer, or more likely to be employed in a job that requires heavy lifting. Moreover, there are probably differences between the two hospitals in the quality of care, the support staff, the equipment available, etc.

Solution: a key aspect of an RCT is that subjects are assigned to receive either the traditional or the new form of surgery, at both hospitals, at random. When the two groups of subjects who received the traditional or new form of surgery are compared, they are likely to be similar. The aim is to make a fair comparison between like groups.

Problem 3: the surgeons claim that 60 per cent of their subjects had a good outcome but how did they decide whether a person did well or not? Might they – or the subjects – have been influenced to say that people were doing better than they really were, so as to portray the surgical procedure in a favourable light?

Solution: RCTs typically involve measuring how well participants do using pre-specified criteria. The outcome measure or end-point of an RCT might be a specially developed questionnaire in which, for example, subjects are asked to rate their level of pain, or it might be a laboratory measurement, such as haemoglobin level, or a combination of these. In some RCTs, assessment is made blind: the researchers assessing the subjects do not know which treatment they received to avoid bias in their assessment.

Problem 4: the surgeons claim that because a 60 per cent success rate is better than 50 per cent, their treatment is more effective. However, if two people have a coin-tossing competition, one could throw more heads purely by chance. Even if they toss 100 coins each, there is about a 15 per cent chance that one will throw at least 10 more heads than the other will.

Solution: the results of RCTs are analysed using statistical methods to determine the probability that there is a **real** difference between treatments, as opposed to any **apparent** benefit being due to chance.

Defining the question

Research is more reliable than personal experience as a basis for general claims or beliefs about health because it is systematically designed to avoid error. This suggests that the way to address beliefs about CAM is through research. Many people believe that conventional medical research has been very successful at improving health: people have much longer and healthier lives today than they did 200 years ago. Although the main cause of this is improved social conditions, medical research has played an important role, which has led to a good understanding of the causes of disease and how to prevent and treat it (Hibberts and MacQueen, 2003).

However, what about CAM? Can it be researched in the same way as conventional medicine? There are some obvious and immediate difficulties. For instance, in the example described above of using rose oil to treat bulimia, a clinical trial was said to be the accepted way to find out whether treatment was effective. A double-blind trial was described in which participants are given either a treatment or an indistinguishable placebo. Devising a placebo for rose oil is relatively straightforward – for example, a base oil containing a synthetic perfume could be used. But what would be the placebo for an aromatherapy massage? It is difficult to give someone a 'mock massage' and there must be a placebo for a double-blind trial. This sort of problem has led many critics to doubt the value of conventional research for CAM. To assess the applicability of 'standard' research methodology to CAM research, it may be necessary to go back to basics: to consider the hypothesis being tested, and modify the methodology so that relevant, appropriate questions can be addressed. The rest of this section describes some of the other standard research protocols that are available, and considers whether any are particularly suitable for CAM research.

Other methodological approaches

The double-blind trial – in which doctors give volunteers either a drug or a placebo and compare how they progress – is only one particular research method, although it is the most highly rated by the scientific research community. However, RCTs and their applications are only suitable for asking particular types of question, such as whether treatments do more harm than good. Many different types of research question can be asked about health and medicine and different research methods have been developed to answer these questions. The scientific community uses other methodological approaches that adhere to the principles of the scientific method, some of which are described below.

Epidemiological research

Epidemiologists try to discover the causes of disease by looking at the whole population rather than individuals. Some of the most important health-related discoveries were made by epidemiological research: for instance, the links between smoking and lung cancer and cholera and dirty drinking water. The two most common types of study are the **cohort study** (sometimes called a prospective study) and the **case-control study** (or retrospective study). The cohort study involves two groups, one of which has been exposed to something that is thought to affect health (for example, second-hand or passive smoking or asbestos). The two groups are then followed to see whether they develop a particular disease (such as lung cancer). The case-control study uses the reverse approach: a group of people who have a particular disease (such as heart disease or lung cancer) are asked about previous exposures (for example, whether they smoke) and their answers are compared with those of a group of people who do not have the disease. It is important to realise that epidemiological studies can only reveal links between events and **not** causes.

Epidemiological methods can also be used to answer questions outside the realm of disease causation. For example, the cohort study is a good way of looking at prognosis: a single group of subjects (rather than two, which is more typical in epidemiological research) is followed over time, and medically relevant events are recorded. For instance, in one study, a group of people were followed for 18 months after surgery for lung cancer. The researchers found that many subjects still experienced pain at the scar site (Katz et al., 1996). This information can be used to advise patients and to help design treatments.

Survey research

Social scientists and psychologists often study behaviours and beliefs through surveys. A random sample of a population is asked a set of questions and the proportion giving each answer is recorded. Surveys are often used to find out what consumers are doing (for example, what proportion of cancer patients use CAM) or what doctors are doing (for example, what proportion refer depressed people to counselling). Surveys can also be used to understand views and beliefs (for example, how young people feel about organ donation). Medical researchers have extended survey methods beyond social research to answer questions about disease prevalence. For example, researchers might interview members of the general public about the symptoms of depression. They might then compare depression rates uncovered by the survey with the number of GP consultations for depression, to determine what proportion of people with depression seek treatment from their GP. A lot of demographic information can be gleaned from official surveys such as the national census.

Laboratory research

Much medical research is done in laboratories. Researchers try to understand the underlying mechanism of disease by studying isolated cells and tissues. Their observations, and subsequent designing and testing of hypotheses, are often the starting point for the development of new therapies. The effects of new drugs and surgical techniques are usually studied first in animals – this is done to comply with the current legislation, as defined in the Medicines Act 1995. Results from laboratory research are rarely directly applicable to people, but they can be used to generate hypotheses for human trials. It is precisely because of its roots in basic laboratory research that the biomedical model of health is so widely accepted by both the medical profession and the general public.

7.4 Using qualitative methods in health research

In the field of medicine and health care, research methods that enable quantification and patterns of causality to be identified have a long and well established tradition. However, they have not gone unchallenged by those who question their inability to embrace a more holistic approach to researching the human condition. Rubinstein et al. (2000) argue that health research should take account of the 'broader context', which includes:

> the wider settings of both space and time. For example, an observed health system should be seen in the context of a wider community and culture, and the requirements of that health system may vary with seasonal variation in disease entities as well. ... For instance, health outcomes may be dependent on a combination of individual factors, provider behaviors, family setting, cultural factors, and the community context.
>
> (Rubinstein et al., 2000, pp. 36–7)

They believe that a more multi-level approach drawing on anthropological methods provides the best way to research the 'intersection of biological, psychological, and social aspects of health and illness' (p. 39). Following on from the social sciences as well as nursing research, there is a growing interest in CAM in using qualitative methods, which also draw on methods used in anthropology.

ACTIVITY   WHAT IS QUALITATIVE RESEARCH?

Allow 5 minutes

What do you think 'qualitative research' means?

Comment

Whereas quantitative methods are designed to standardise data so that they can be given a number and measured, qualitative methods are designed to help researchers capture and understand social phenomena in their natural contexts rather than in experimental settings. Qualitative research typically emphasises people's words and actions rather than quantification and measurement. Therefore, qualitative methods strongly emphasise the exploration of people's meanings, definitions, understandings and experiences within their social and cultural context.

Quantitative methods are generally associated with **deductive** reasoning, whereas qualitative methods are generally associated with **inductive** reasoning. The difference between them is that deduction involves a process of data collection in order to **test a theory** or hypothesis, whereas induction involves a process of data collection in order to **generate theories** and generalisations. These newly emerging theories are then 'grounded' by collecting more data to establish whether and to what extent the developing generalisations and theories are accurate and applicable in different circumstances. Typically, research participants' own categories, concepts and meanings are used because it is important to discover what meanings phenomena have for people and what are people's own understandings and interpretations of phenomena. The very nature of the scientific method and quantitative techniques of data gathering means that they are regarded as inadequate for research that aims at grasping the meanings that people attach to phenomena.

Sheila Payne (1997) discusses nursing research which has been particularly concerned to use qualitative methods to research nursing interventions. She draws on the work of Lincoln and Guba (1985) to identify five different assumptions underlying qualitative methods:

1   The nature of reality within the quantitative paradigm is assumed to be single, tangible and fragmentable, while in qualitative research it is believed to be multiple and socially constructed.

2   The role of researcher and researched is clearly defined and independent in quantitative studies rather than interactive. What is more, the researcher is more powerful than the respondent.

3   Quantitative research aims to make generalizations at a population level which are temporally and contextually free, while qualitative researchers emphasize the embeddedness of their results.

4   Quantitative research aims to discover causal mechanisms which are largely conceptualized as linear, while qualitative paradigms emphasize the interactive nature of causality.

5   Finally, the ideal of 'scientific' research is that it is value free and that well planned, careful studies will enable the 'facts' to be discovered. An alternative proposal is that all research is inherently value bound, both in its design and execution, but that the values of the researcher should be presented to readers so that they may use this information in evaluating the study.

(Payne, 1997, p. 105)

The main qualitative research methods

The main techniques of data collection used in qualitative research are participant observation, unstructured and semi-structured interviews, biographical interviews and focus groups, each of which is discussed below.

Participant observation

Observation involves watching people's behaviour and listening to people talk as they interact in their natural setting. This method is based on anthropological techniques but can be used in all types of social settings. It has been used extensively in nursing to research hospitals and other health care settings. Raymond Gold's classification of observational roles is the classic typology for qualitative researchers who use observational methods (Gold, 1958). The extent to which the researcher is detached or involved in what is being observed is integral to Gold's classification. The spectrum of involvement can range from full participation at one end to observer only at the other:

| full participant – participant as observer – observer as participant – observer only. |

The full participant role implies that the observation is covert and not made explicit to the people involved in the setting. It is the role adopted by undercover agents and investigative journalists and clearly has ethical problems for health care research. However, it has the benefit of being able to observe behaviour which is not specially adapted for the researchers. The middle two roles are more appropriate to health care settings. The participant as observer role can be typified in nursing research by a nurse who works in a particular setting as a nurse but is also doing research. The observational role is known to everyone else in the setting, including the patients. The observer as participant role applies where the researcher is there primarily in a research capacity but, in order to blend into the surroundings, performs tasks and helps out generally. Researchers who are participant-observers make copious notes about their observations when and how they can – in coffee breaks, in lunch breaks and at the end of a shift – but rarely while observing, so as not to influence what is going on. The pure observer role at the other end of the spectrum is less concerned with being unobtrusive and can record when and how events happen. Participant-observers also augment their observational data with interviews, as described below.

Unstructured and semi-structured interviews

These are usually face-to-face and aim to explore topics in detail. They are often called 'in-depth' interviews because they enable the researcher to access in-depth details. Typically, in-depth interviews are not structured by a list of predefined questions that the researcher wants to ask. In semi-structured interviews the researcher may have a checklist or an interview guide of topics they would like to cover. In unstructured interviews the researcher may have just a list of prompts to help their memory and this type of interview is much more like a conversation. These types of interview are very flexible because the idea is that, within the relevant subject area of the research, the researcher encourages the interviewee to talk about matters that are important or relevant to the interviewee. As far as possible, the researcher attempts to gather data that will enable them to see the interviewee's point of view, which avoids imposing the researcher's own categories of interest or those the researcher assumes are important to the interviewee.

Biographical or life-history interviews

These draw on the respondents' past experiences to illuminate their present circumstances. These types of interview have been used to good effect in understanding the health status and needs of older people (Sidell, 1998).

Focus groups

This is a method of interviewing groups of people about predefined topics. In general, the researcher selects focus-group interviewees because their views or experiences are judged by the researcher to be useful for exploring the research issues. Focus-group interviewing explicitly involves encouraging interviewees to interact in discussing the topics because this interaction can generate information about how people jointly construct meanings and share understandings about phenomena.

Qualitative researchers often use a combination of research methods or sources of data to study something as a way to check the validity of their findings. This use of multiple methods and data sources is known as **triangulation** and is also frequently associated with quantitative work.

Uses of qualitative research

Some research methods are better suited than others to investigating different types of research question. Pope and Mays (1995) argue that as medicine and health provision advance, health and health services becomes a more diverse and complex arena in which increasing numbers of research questions arise that cannot be adequately explored by quantitative methods. They argue that health care deals with people, and people are generally a more complex subject for investigation than the subject matter investigated by the natural sciences. Hence, researching health care is likely to involve researching questions about human interaction and interpretations for which experimental and quantitative methods are inappropriate. For example, as genetic technology advances, people are faced with making unprecedented decisions about reproduction or the predisposition to or transmission of genetic diseases. Therefore, it is important to try to understand how and why people conceptualise genetic risks and why they behave in the way they do when faced with these risks (Pope and Mays, 1995). Semi-structured or unstructured interviewing by a sensitive and skilled interviewer is highly suitable for researching these issues because it enables subtle nuances and shades of meaning to be drawn out in a way that quantitative methods are less well suited to do.

Although qualitative and quantitative methods are often portrayed as opposing research approaches and, in the medical field, the validity and rigour of qualitative methods are still questioned, studies are now appearing in medical journals that demonstrate a full awareness of the specificity of qualitative methods (Borreani et al., 2004).

There are several ways of using qualitative methods to research medicine and health care. Pope and Mays (1995) note three ways in which qualitative methods can complement quantitative work.

1   A preliminary stage of quantitative work: for example, observation or interviews can be used to establish an understanding of an event, a situation or a behaviour or to discover the most comprehensible terms and words to use in a subsequent questionnaire.

2   A supplement to quantitative work: for example, a questionnaire may uncover one version of respondents' beliefs and attitudes, but observation and in-depth interviewing on the same topic may reveal that respondents hold more private, complex or contradictory views than were elicited by the pre-set questions in the questionnaire.

3   To explore complex areas that are unsuited to quantitative methods, such as both the declared and the tacit routines and rules used by doctors in clinical decision making.

7.5   What constitutes evidence in CAM research?

The philosophical notion which the biomedical model is based on is usually considered to be 'reductionism'. This perspective reduces phenomena, including those relating to the body, to their constituent parts and seeks to establish one-dimensional, linear, causal relationships between variables that can be expressed in quantified, statistical terms. The philosophical approach of CAM is founded on the notion of 'holism', which means the nature of CAM interventions is based on a philosophical understanding of the complete person in terms of mind, body, spirit and lifestyle. Advocates of CAM are concerned that the nature of a CAM healing experience is located in a different world view of health and healing which is not amenable to the views and methods of orthodox medical research. Therefore, research on CAM should be done in a different manner using different methods.

Does 'alternative medicine' require 'alternative research'?

In the 1980s and early 1990s an active debate continued about whether conventional research methods were appropriate for CAM. Some supporters of CAM were vigorously opposed to the use of conventional methodology, even going so far as to claim that it would constitute 'acts of epistemological violence' (Scheid, 1993). Some of these radical opinions are listed in Box 7.3 (overleaf).

There were two main areas of concern. First, science was seen as impersonal and mechanistic, which did not seem to fit well with the intimate and emotional aspects of many CAM treatments such as massage or meditation (see arguments 1 and 2 in Box 7.3). Second, it was thought that doing conventional research on CAM therapies would involve changing the therapies in some way, destroying their true nature and turning them into a form of orthodox medicine (see quotations 3 and 4). One explanation for these bold statements is that CAM advocates are really most concerned about RCTs, the gold standard used in conventional medicine for determining whether a treatment is effective. However, even though CAM use is sometimes aimed more at improving general wellbeing

> **BOX 7.3   ARGUMENTS AGAINST THE USE OF CONVENTIONAL RESEARCH TO EVALUATE CAM**
>
> 1 Scientific advancement 'is an aggressive, invasive form of probing, dissection and analysis into a soul-less world of space, time, matter and forces [in which] a human being [becomes] an accidental arrangement of molecules in an impersonal "dead" universe' (St George, 1994a, p. 255).
>
> 2 Conventional research is a tool for regulating the development of an illness, something which requires a passive body and the use of treatments which maintain that passivity (Launsø, 1995).
>
> 3 'Those of us concerned with protecting [CAM] therapies from unnecessary encroachment and control ... [require] new models of research' (Mills, 1986, p. 42).
>
> 4 Conventional research 'requires a complete submission to the orthodox medical paradigm', possibly leading 'to the take-over of complementary medicine by orthodox doctors' and 'a distortion of its essential nature in order to ... fit into the needs and vested interests of orthodox medicine' (St George, 1994b, p. 38).

than at curing a specific ailment, such issues can still be elucidated by other methods. There are other methodologies which have validity in the research culture and which are, perhaps, more applicable to CAM research.

Evidence of efficacy: challenging RCTs

The use of RCTs to produce rigorous evidence for the efficacy of CAM is greatly challenged in some parts of the CAM world for several reasons.

Conventionally, the efficacy of treatments was determined by assessing the progression of symptoms or by monitoring the functioning of organs through the use of quantitative methods. However, Kelner and Wellman (2003) argue that the concept of what constitutes evidence of efficacy should be expanded because different groups of people use different types of evidence. For example, consumers of CAM consider efficacy in terms of their overall health and wellbeing and tend to use a variety of types of evidence when making decisions about their use of CAM. Consumers treat these different types of evidence as valid and legitimate, although they may not be formally recognised as rigorous evidence by the scientific community.

ACTIVITY   DIFFERENT TYPES OF EVIDENCE

Allow 30 minutes

What sources and types of information might people use as 'evidence' of efficacy to help them make decisions about using CAM? You may have had your own experiences of using different types of information to help you make decisions about using CAM or you may know about the information that other people used to make their decisions.

Comment

What constitutes acceptable, legitimate evidence is not the same for everyone. When making decisions about their health care, people can rely on or be influenced by many different types of information from a variety of sources. Kelner and Wellman (2003) argue that the research indicates few people who decide to use CAM were recommended to it by their physicians. People tend to be most influenced by recommendations from people they trust who have benefited from CAM, such as family or friends. As well as relying on advice from these 'health confidants', people are also influenced by:

- information from work colleagues, acquaintances and CAM practitioners

- media reports of successful CAM use

- advertisements for CAM, for example in specialised publications, health food outlets and in the mainstream media

- internet sources of information on health knowledge and advice.

Kelner and Wellman argue that, since the outcome of the healing process is also influenced by several factors – such as the therapeutic relationship, the practitioner's intuition and experience and the patient's confidence and participation – a variety of different types of evidence should be considered in evaluating the efficacy of CAM.

Advocates of CAM – for example, Verhoef et al. (2002) and Kelner and Wellman (2003) – are concerned about the following issues.

- It is difficult or impossible to conduct RCTs on many CAM modalities adequately because finding appropriate placebos and ensuring blinding are very difficult. For example, how could a placebo massage be given and how can people be tested blind in a trial of meditation?
- A typical feature of RCTs is that standardised treatment is measured for everyone with a particular diagnosis. This standardisation makes RCTs inappropriate for CAM interventions, which are specifically tailored for each individual and may use several modalities simultaneously (co-interventions). CAM interventions may also be adjusted or changed during a course of treatment. Furthermore, there may be a variety of ways

in which some CAM therapies are delivered: for example, chiropractic can be practised in different ways. Thus, the RCT method of research is unlikely to adequately address these variations.

■ Defining clinical problems or hypotheses to be tested by RCTs may be difficult. CAM interventions often apply to non-specific conditions such as stress or low energy and, rather than treating specific conditions, CAM interventions often invoke concepts that are not recognised by biomedicine, such as 'body energy' and 'restoring balance to the body'.

■ Recruiting people and randomly allocating them for RCTs in CAM may prove difficult because people's beliefs, practices and preferences vary widely.

■ RCTs attempt to minimise the impact of personal experience (non-specific factors) on the outcomes of the trial. Mercer et al. (1995) suggest that it is better to use objective outcomes based on medical criteria rather than patients' own accounts. This is a problem because CAM advocates and practitioners consider clients' subjective reports to be highly relevant and, further, that the therapeutic effect of the practitioner–client relationship is crucial and integral to the CAM intervention.

Advocates of RCTs have attempted to address the objections of CAM advocates. For example, Vickers (1996) suggests that RCTs are clearly not necessarily based on a reductionist linear causal view since there have been RCTs of phenomena such as psychotherapy and prayer. He argues that RCTs researching psychotherapy consist of an interactive dialogue between practitioner and patient, and thus cannot be seen as linear, and that RCTs on prayer are unlikely to either reduce the whole to its constituent parts or assume mechanistic causality. Vickers also argues that RCTs do not claim to be able to explain complex causal relationships between variables: they only determine whether such a relationship exists. For example, does psychotherapy reliably change a person's health status, such as giving relief from emotional distress? In response to some of the concerns about RCTs, Vickers argues that placebos and blinding are not needed to carry out an RCT. For example, the standard treatment rather than a placebo may be used with the control group and, in trials involving follow-ups, practitioners or users generally know that follow-ups have happened. RCT treatments do not need to be standardised and measurable either. Although drugs and doses are normally standardised in drug therapy RCTs, many other areas of medicine cannot be reduced to a 'single treatment formula' and RCTs can be used to compare different models of a treatment. Further, objective outcome measures are not a requirement of RCTs, many of which rely exclusively on patients' reports.

In order to address the shortcomings of RCTs, there is growing interest in **pragmatic trials**. This adaptation of RCTs allows experimental clinical trials to be undertaken in ways that retain, as far as possible, the natural context in which practice is carried out, thus eliminating the need for double-blinding, placebos, standardised treatments or objective outcomes (Vickers, 1996; Verhoef et al., 2002).

Evidence for the safety of CAM

CAM therapies are widely believed to be perfectly safe because of their long history of use. In fact, this perceived safety is one of the commonest reasons why people choose CAM modalities instead of conventional therapies. What they often forget – or ignore – is that, first, by no means all modalities have a long history of use and, second, until recently there has rarely been any systematic reporting of the negative effects of CAM therapies. More worryingly, data about safety are scarce for particular groups, such as pregnant women, children or older people. So what is the real story about the safety of CAM modalities? Are there grounds for answering 'yes' to the fundamental question 'Does this therapy do more good than harm'? If so, is there a case for using RCTs?

There is some justification for homeopaths to claim that their treatments cannot harm because they are so highly diluted. However, in about 20 per cent of treatments the symptoms worsen, which practitioners believe indicates that the treatment is working. Nevertheless, it is a drawback for the patient (Grabia and Ernst, 2003). Also, cases of allergic reaction have been reported with remedies that are not highly diluted (Ernst et al., 2001).

Acupuncture has a long history of use and is relatively free of reported adverse effects. There have been some serious, adverse events, mainly because dirty needles were used, including septicaemia and hepatitis B infections. However, a large study by a Japanese acupuncture clinic, in which they followed up all their patients over a five-year period, revealed only 64 adverse effects from several thousand patients. This suggests that acupuncture is a fairly safe procedure when properly carried out but that issues of practitioner competence may be important (Yamashita et al., 1998)

Herbal medicine presents more of a problem. It is no coincidence that a majority of today's conventional drugs are derived from plant products. Plants contain numerous, highly biologically active compounds, many of which can affect people in unexpected ways, yet most herbal remedies are exempt from testing and product licensing under the Medicines Act 1968. Although pure extracts can be characterised and their biological and toxicological properties rigorously assessed, a major problem with herbal medicine is the unreliability of source materials (Schultz et al., 2000). Apparently similar doses can actually contain widely differing amounts of the active substance, and there are many instances of contamination with several substances ranging from microbial toxins to herbicides. Even more worryingly, many herbal medicines can interact with other drugs that the patient may be taking. The interactions of St John's Wort with conventional anti-depressants and oral contraceptives are well known (Barnes, 2003); perhaps less widely known are the possible interactions of herbal remedies with 'mild' drugs such as aspirin (Elvin-Lewis, 2001).

There is a basic need to reassure the public that herbal remedies are at least safe, whatever other claims can or cannot be made for their effectiveness. While arguing for a broader range of ways of investigating effectiveness, reassurance about safety can only come from adhering to research methods that are tried and tested within the scientific paradigm. As Simon Mills points out:

> the licence to market herbs as medicines for what are considered moderate to severe conditions is dependent on providing conventional clinical evidence for such a claim. The double-blind clinical trials and experiments on animals, to name two areas of contention in research, will remain essential as evidence as long as legislative and medical authorities consider them so.
>
> (Mills, 1991, pp. 238–9)

To research the whole CAM experience in terms of both efficacy and safety clearly requires a combination of research methodologies which encompass the quantitative scientific method and more qualitative approaches.

7.6   Combining methods in researching CAM

As noted in Section 7.5, RCTs mainly produce general, aggregated forms of knowledge about the frequency and the strength of any causal relationships, so their use for researching the efficacy of CAM is contested. Verhoef et al. (2002) propose that this problem can be overcome by adding qualitative methods to RCT research, so that specific information can be captured about the why and the how of individual CAM experiences. For example, an RCT may show that a treatment had no effect in terms of the hypothesis, but it will not show whether the treatment worked in other ways and whether some people benefited. So, qualitative interviews may be used, which could reveal that some people thought there was a change in their health after treatment, such as a greater feeling of relaxation or an increase in energy. These changes may not be recognised as 'improvement' by the outcome measures used in an RCT, so qualitative interviewing can be used to detect other potential benefits of CAM treatment that cannot be detected by the RCT.

Verhoef et al. (2002) also argue that qualitative methods are particularly useful for researching CAM treatments because they enable the exploration of people's meanings, purpose and spirituality in the context of the whole life and being of the individual. As discussed in Section 7.2, this is particularly relevant in holism and the strong belief in many CAM modalities that the mind cannot be separated from the body.

Following their call for the inclusion of a variety of types of evidence in CAM evaluations (see the activity in Section 7.5), Kelner and Wellman (2003) also advocate the use of both qualitative and quantitative methods of research. They argue that both methods are necessary because each one emphasises different world views, or aspects of reality, recognising the 'complex interplay of biological, psychological, social, cultural, environmental and spiritual factors underlying health and disease' (p. 23).

Although RCTs are used to research CAM, concerns continue about their ability to capture and evaluate the holistic experience of CAM treatment. Ribeaux and Spence (2001) highlight a major problem: that the more holistic the CAM approach is, the more difficult it is to evaluate its efficacy through RCTs because what is implied is 'an ever increasing range of inter-therapist and inter-patient differences' (p. 190). They argue that questions such as 'Does aromatherapy work for lower back pain?' are inappropriate because the answer depends on who the practitioner is, the quality of their touch and what other skills they use. To resolve this problem, the authors advocate that a more appropriate research question is one that evaluates the practitioner rather than the treatment, since treatments and therapies are put together for individual people by the practitioner.

Ribeaux and Spence (2001) also advocate the use of both qualitative and quantitative methods to study the process and the outcomes of the therapeutic intervention. Qualitative methods are ideally suited to identify the 'active ingredients' in the CAM intervention and how they interact. The authors suggest that several interventions by different practitioners with different people could be observed by using video cameras or two-way mirrors. The treatment delivery should be observed as it happens in its natural context. Interpreting the significance of the observations of the treatment process could be aided by follow-up interviews with practitioners, and interviews or focus groups with clients or users, so that interpretations are as close as possible to their perspective. Holistic measures of the treatment outcome could then be devised, expressed in the words of practitioners and patients, and these measures could be used to identify some of the main dimensions involved in holism, including dimensions that distinguish effective from ineffective practitioners.

Ribeaux and Spence go on to argue that this move of emphasis away from the intervention and towards the practitioner applies to both CAM and orthodox medicine. They maintain that such a move 'serves a number of purposes: 1) it enables some kind of resolution of the reductionism/holism debate; 2) it puts conventional medicine and CAM on the same playing field; and 3) it retains the rigour of the scientific methods in evaluation trials' (p. 192). Ribeaux and Spence's views are explored further in Chapter 9.

7.7   Conclusion

This chapter introduced several important issues and debates that influence people's understanding of what research is and how it should be done in the fields of biomedicine and CAM.

Much research in orthodox medicine is focused on producing evidence through studies using the principles of the scientific method. However, there is growing interest in biomedicine in using qualitative methods to investigate the increasing numbers of health questions that require an understanding of the subtle nuances of human interaction.

In the field of CAM there is active debate about whether the research standards and methods used in biomedical research are appropriate for researching CAM. A particular concern of CAM advocates is whether the use of RCTs is appropriate for determining the efficacy of CAM modalities.

KEY POINTS

- There are contested views about what the form and nature of phenomena are, which are often referred to as world views or perspectives.

- There are contested theories about what 'knowledge' is because different perspectives on the form and nature of phenomena influence people's understanding of what constitutes valid, legitimate knowledge about them.

- Biomedicine and biomedical research are frequently associated with a 'reductionist' world view, which involves reducing phenomena or processes to their constituent parts in order to analyse them and the relationships between them. This world view usually emphasises objective measures and quantitative methods of research.

- Current biomedical perspectives on what constitutes valid, legitimate research and evidence are usually based on the principles of the 'scientific method', which involves following a set of clearly defined, systematic, replicable steps to test hypotheses. Randomised controlled trials (RCTs) are probably the most well known type of medical research in this world view.

- The use of qualitative methods for researching areas of concern to biomedicine is gaining popularity. Developments and expansion in medicine and health care mean that now many more types of questions are arising that are not easily investigated by experimental, quantitative methods of research. Qualitative methods can also be used to inform the development of quantitative work and to supplement it.

- CAM therapies are associated with a 'holistic' world view of health in which the social, spiritual and physical aspects of an individual are inseparable. Advocates of CAM question whether and to what extent the research standards and techniques used in biomedical research are appropriate for researching CAM because the nature of a CAM healing experience is located in a different world view of health and healing.

- Many advocates of CAM are concerned that the use of RCTs alone for determining the efficacy of CAM therapies is inappropriate because they focus on a limited concept of what constitutes efficacy.

- These advocates of CAM argue for the use of both qualitative and quantitative methods in researching CAM treatments and outcomes. Qualitative methods enable the exploration of how people experience phenomena and make sense of them in their life context. This type of information is highly relevant in a holistic view of health and health care.

References

Banting, F. C. (1925, published 1965) 'Nobel Lecture', in *Nobel Lectures: Physiology or Medicine, 1922–1941*, Amsterdam, Elsevier.

Barnes, J. (2003) 'Quality, efficacy and safety of complementary medicines: fashions, facts and the future. Part II: Efficacy and safety', *British Journal of Clinical Pharmacology*, Vol. 55, pp. 331–40.

Borreani, C., Miccinesi, G., Brunelli, C. and Lina, M. (2004) 'An increasing number of qualitative research papers in oncology and palliative care: does it mean a thorough development of the methodology of research?', *Health and Quality of Life Outcomes*, Vol. 2, No. 7. Available online at: www.hqlo.com/content/2/1/7 [accessed 24 January 2005].

Czyz, J., Nikolova, T., Schuderer, J., Kuster, N. and Wobus, A. M. (2004) 'Non-thermal effects of power-line magnetic fields (50 Hz) on gene expression levels of pluripotent embryonic stem cells – the role of tumour suppressor', *Mutation Research*, Vol. 557, pp. 63–74.

Elvin-Lewis, M. (2001) 'Should we be concerned about herbal remedies?', *Journal of Ethnopharmacology*, Vol. 75, pp. 141–64.

Ernst, E., Pittler, M. H., Stevinson, C. and White, A. (2001) *The Desktop Guide to Complementary and Alternative Medicine*, London, Mosby.

Gold, R. L. (1958) 'Roles in sociological field observations', *Social Forces*, Vol. 36, No. 3, pp. 217–23.

Grabia, S. and Ernst, E. (2003) 'Homeopathic aggravations: a systematic review of randomised, placebo-controlled clinical trials', *Homoeopathy*, Vol. 92, pp. 92–8.

Hibberts, L. and MacQueen, H. (2003) *Diagnosing Infection*, Book 4 of S320 Infectious Disease, Milton Keynes, The Open University.

Katz, J., Jackson, M., Kavanagh, B. P. and Sandler, A. N. (1996) 'Acute pain after thoracic surgery predicts long-term post-thoracotomy pain', *Clinical Journal of Pain*, Vol. 12, pp. 50–55.

Kelner, M. and Wellman, B. (2003) 'Complementary and alternative medicine: how do we know if it works?', *Healthcare Papers*, Vol. 3, No. 5, pp. 10–28.

Kettler, H. (2001) *Consolidation and Competition in the Pharmaceutical Industry*, London, Office of Health Economics.

Launsø, L. (1995) 'How to kiss a monster', in Johannessen, H. et al. (eds) *Studies in Alternative Therapy 1*, Denmark, Odense University Press.

Leask, J. and McIntyre, P. (2003) 'Public opponents of vaccination: a case study', *Vaccine*, Vol. 21, pp. 4700–3.

Lincoln, Y. S. and Guba, E. G. (1985) *Naturalistic Inquiry*, Beverly Hills, CA, Sage.

Mercer, G., Long, A. F. and Smith, I. J. (1995) *Researching and Evaluating Complementary Therapies: The State of the Debate*, Leeds, Nuffield Institute for Health.

Mills, S. (1986) 'Conflicting research needs in complementary medicine', *Complementary Medicine Research*, Vol. 1, No. 1, pp. 40–7.

Mills, S. Y. (1991) *The Essential Book of Herbal Medicine*, London, Arkana/ Penguin.

Payne, S. (1997) 'Nursing research: a social science?', in McKenzie, G., Powell, J. and Usher, R. (eds) *Understanding Social Research: Perspectives on Methodology and Practice*, pp. 101–12, London, Falmer Press.

Pope, C. and Mays, N. (1995) 'Qualitative research: reaching the parts other methods cannot reach: an introduction to qualitative methods in health and health services research', *British Medical Journal*, Vol. 311, pp. 42–45.

Popper, K. (1959) *The Logic of Scientific Discovery*, New York, Basic Books.

Ribeaux, P. and Spence, M. (2001) 'CAM evaluation: what are the research questions?', *Complementary Therapies in Medicine*, Vol. 9, pp. 188–93.

Rubinstein, R. A., Scrimshaw, S. C. and Morrissey, S. E. (2000) 'Classification and process in sociomedical understanding: towards a multilevel view of sociomedical methodology', in Albrecht, G. L., Fitzpatrick, R. and Scrimshaw, S. C. (eds) *The Handbook of Social Studies in Health and Medicine*, pp. 36–49, London, Sage.

Sackett, D., Rosenberg, W., Gray, J., Haynes, R. and Richardson, W. (1996) 'Evidence based medicine: what it is and what it isn't', *British Medical Journal*, Vol. 312, pp. 71–2.

Scheid, V. (1993) 'Orientalism revisited', *European Journal of Oriental Medicine*, Vol. 1, No. 2, pp. 23–33.

Schultz, V., Hänsel, R. and Tyler, V. E. (2000) *Rational Phytotherapy. A Physician's Guide to Herbal Medicine* (4th edition), Berlin, Springer.

Sidell, M. (1998) 'Treatment or tender loving care?', in Brechin, A., Walmsley, J., Katz, J. and Peace, S. (eds) *Care Matters: Concepts, Practice and Research in Health and Social Care*, pp. 96–106, London, Sage.

Silverman, W. A. and Chalmers, I. (2001) 'Casting and drawing lots: a time honoured way of dealing with uncertainty and ensuring fairness', *British Medical Journal*, Vol. 323, pp. 1467–8.

St George, D. (1994a) 'Towards a research and development strategy for complementary medicine', *The Homeopath*, Vol. 54, pp. 254–6.

St George, D. (1994b) 'Research and development in herbal medicine: biomedical research or new paradigm?', *European Journal of Herbal Medicine*, Vol. 1, No. 1, pp. 38–40.

Verhoef, M. J., Casebeer, A. L. and Hilsden, R. J. (2002) 'Assessing efficacy of complementary medicine: adding qualitative methods to the "Gold Standard"', *The Journal of Alternative and Complementary Medicine*, Vol. 8, No. 3, pp. 275–81.

Vickers, A. (1996) 'Methodological issues in complementary and alternative medicine research: a personal reflection on 10 years of debate in the United Kingdom', *The Journal of Alternative and Complementary Medicine*, Vol. 2, No. 4, pp. 515–24.

World Medical Association (2000) *Declaration of Helsinki* [online], www.wma.net/e/ethicsunit/helsinki.htm [accessed 24 January 2005].

Yamashita, H., Tsukayama, J., Tanno, Y. and Nishijo, K. (1998) 'Adverse effects related to acupuncture', *Journal of the American Medical Association*, Vol. 280, pp. 1563–4.

Chapter 8 Researching CAM interventions

Tom Heller

Contents

AIMS

- To describe the ways in which different types of CAM-related research can be used to demonstrate the effectiveness of CAM.
- To give an insight into the variety of research methodologies that can be used to study CAM.

8.1 Introduction

Chapters 6 and 7 discussed how research can investigate a wide range of questions. In this chapter the focus moves specifically to some of the ways of researching interventions in complementary and alternative medicine (CAM). 'Research' findings can be used by different interest groups to promote their own interests. Research is used for highly political and for economic purposes in advertisements, or to promote certain points of view. Commercial ventures may make claims based on 'research': for example, to sell particular CAM services or products. However, the debate running throughout this book, particularly in Chapter 7, is how best to research CAM interventions: in other words, which research methods are appropriate to researching CAM?

The 'gold standard' of research methodology favoured by biomedicine traditionally is the scientific method. This includes randomised controlled trials (RCTs), experiments and surveys, all of which are quantifiable, providing statistical data that can be generalised. Given the dominance of biomedicine in the health field, CAM researchers have been expected to prove its effectiveness using the research techniques that are acceptable to biomedicine. Many CAM modalities, especially those wanting statutory regulatory and professional status, and possible integration within the National Health Service (NHS), have embraced the scientific method. However, other CAM modalities are opposed to this on the grounds that the scientific method is 'reductionist' in its approach to health matters and so is at odds with the philosophical principle of most CAM modalities – 'holism' (see Chapter 7).

A glimpse of the current state of CAM research reveals a lot of activity using orthodox scientific methods but also a growing literature of dissent. This advocates the use of more qualitative methods which, it is argued, can delve deeper into the complex nature of CAM and engage with the CAM experience in a holistic way. The way forward for many is to combine the more quantifiable orthodox scientific methods with qualitative methods. This will then provide evidence which is objective and capable of statistical analysis and generalisation, as well as evidence that reveals the depth and complexity of people's subjective experiences of CAM.

To give a flavour of CAM research, several examples of published research were selected for this chapter. These examples use various techniques to answer specific research questions. The different reports of the research demonstrate certain features of current research methodology – some quantitative, some qualitative. They illustrate the dilemmas inherent in building a research base for CAM that will both satisfy biomedical criteria and be true to the philosophical foundations of CAM. The first four cases in Section 8.2 are examples of research within the orthodox scientific paradigm. Section 8.3 discusses two systematic reviews of several studies on the same topic but still within the quantitative tradition. Section 8.4 moves on to examine examples of qualitative research and Section 8.5 gives examples of combining qualitative and quantitative methods to illuminate CAM practice.

8.2   Working within the 'gold standard'

Many thousands of CAM research studies have used orthodox research methods. In June 2003, the medical database MedLine listed 67,000 papers on CAM, about 3000 of which were RCTs. Many of these RCTs have provided useful information. For example, it is now 'known' that: hypnosis and relaxation techniques can help cancer patients (Anon., 1996); acupuncture is probably beneficial for headaches, but does not help people quit smoking (Linde et al., 2001); and chiropractic can be helpful for back pain (Meade et al., 1990). In addition, some of the non-RCTs have revealed potentially significant findings. For example, a cohort study found that cancer patients who have unusual alternative cancer treatments may have shorter survival times compared with patients who do not use such methods (Risberg et al., 2002). Surveys have reported how widespread CAM use is, and how most patients use CAM in addition to, rather than instead of, conventional medicine (Eisenberg et al., 1998). Animal studies have started to uncover some of the biological explanations for why acupuncture might be effective (Stux and Hammerschlag, 2000). Laboratory studies are also showing why some herbs might be active against cancer, leading to the development of new combinations of conventional and herbal treatments (Cheung et al., 2002). There seems to be a growing body of well designed and executed, rigorously analysed and realistically interpreted evidence of the efficacy of some CAM modalities for treating certain conditions. The case studies and associated activities in this chapter will guide you through the research maze.

Case Study 1: Is aromatherapy a safe and effective treatment for managing agitation in people with severe dementia?

In this case study a double-blind, placebo-controlled trial was used to study people with a confirmed diagnosis (severe dementia) in order to evaluate the effectiveness of a specific CAM intervention – aromatherapy with *Melissa officinalis* or lemon balm. Two of the major features of this research are that a 'control' group was used and that this group was given a form of treatment that was similar to the 'active' treatment. The people administering the therapy to both groups were apparently not aware whether they were giving the active treatment or the control treatment: 'double-blind' refers to both the people who received the treatment and the people administering it. The researchers also attempted to make objective observations of the outcomes of the different types of treatment in both groups.

It can be difficult to 'blind' CAM studies:

> how could a treatment such as acupuncture or chiropractic manipulation be delivered without the patient knowing whether they were receiving it or not? Since many CAM treatments do not involve taking pills, it is very difficult to devise placebo controls for CAM interventions.

> (Grimm, 2002, p. 145)

However, some investigators have worked to develop 'sham' or placebo controls that can be used in research as the 'control arm' against which to compare 'active' types of treatment. In homeopathy and herbalism, the use of placebo medication is comparatively straightforward and researchers looking for sham acupuncture techniques have been particularly resourceful (Filshie and Cummings, 1999).

The existence of 'the placebo effect' calls into question the validity of such research (Di Blasi, 2003). (The 'placebo effect' was discussed in Chapter 6.) It happens when research participants seem to improve although they were given 'merely a placebo' and not the treatment being tested. Di Blasi argues that 'the placebo effect' indicates that there can be powerful psychological processes at work when people receive treatment. Similarly, many CAM practitioners argue that it is not only the treatment that people receive that affects the outcome: it is how it is delivered. CAM enthusiasts and therapists insist that the imposition of comparatively rigid 'scientific' research is not appropriate to the study of the holistic nature of much CAM practice. Discussion about the usefulness of transferring this type of 'scientific' testing into the CAM world continues (Margolin et al., 1998; Ernst, 2002).

This type of research is comparatively common in the field of orthodox medicine where many different therapies, particularly drugs, are tested against each other, and often against control groups which have no active therapy. Indeed, this is a prerequisite for introducing new types of therapy into the orthodox medical system.

ACTIVITY   A DOUBLE-BLIND, PLACEBO-CONTROLLED STUDY

Allow 30 minutes

Read the description in Box 8.1 of research published by Clive Ballard and his colleagues in the UK (Ballard et al., 2002). As you read, make notes in answer to the following questions.

1   What problems do you think might have arisen out of the attempt to 'double-blind' this research?

2   Can you think of any ethical issues that might arise in research of this nature?

BOX 8.1   MELISSA AROMATHERAPY IN THE TREATMENT OF PEOPLE WITH DEMENTIA

Background

In an increasingly elderly population the numbers of people with dementia can be expected to rise. The usual focus of public and professional attention is on the cognitive problems that people with dementia face. However, more than 50 per cent of people with dementia also experience 'behavioural or psychological symptoms in dementia' (BPSDs; Finkel et al., 2000). These symptoms are problematic for the people with dementia and their carers. In addition, they are difficult to treat with the available range of mood-altering drugs (Burns et al., 2002). The most problematic BPSD in people with dementia is probably agitation, which may be particularly amenable to certain types of aromatherapy.

Aromatherapy, which uses extracts of plants and other 'essential oils', has a long history of helping people who are agitated, restless or feeling low.

Melissa, or lemon balm, is one plant species that has been associated with this form of aromatherapy targeted at behavioural problems.

Research hypothesis

Using melissa as part of aromatherapy treatment would result in an improvement in the symptoms of agitation experienced by people with severe dementia, compared with the use of a placebo, and result in benefits to the quality of life of people within the study.

Method

A total of 72 people living in eight NHS nursing homes were the subjects of the study. Half of them (36) received the active treatment and the other half received a placebo. All these people had a diagnosis of severe dementia and displayed features of agitation including anxiety, irritability, wandering, aggression, shouting and night-time disturbances. These behaviours were measured serially using various validated measures, including the Cohen-Mansfield Agitation Inventory. In addition, Dementia Care Mapping (DCM) was used to provide an objective measure of quality of life. This technique is an observational measure during which people's activities and behaviours are measured every five minutes over a six-hour period (Kitwood and Bredin, 1992). For all participants, DCM assessments were repeated at weekly intervals over the four-week study period. Neither the carers, residents nor people carrying out the assessments were aware of which participants were receiving the melissa therapy and which were getting the placebo.

The active treatment lotion was made of melissa oil and a base lotion; the placebo lotion contained sunflower oil and the base lotion. The lotion was applied twice each day by care assistants to the face and arms of all the people in the study. Each treatment took between 1 and 2 minutes.

Results

A total of 71 people completed the trial (one person died during the period of the research from entirely unrelated causes). Five people (two in the active group and three in the placebo group) were prescribed additional medication for behavioural symptoms during the trial.

- **Changes in agitation** On the standardised agitation scale, mean improvements of 35 per cent were seen on active treatment, compared with 11 per cent on placebo. This is a significant difference.
- **Changes in quality of life** Among people receiving active treatment, there was a significant reduction in the percentage of time spent socially withdrawn, and a significant increase in the percentage of time engaged in constructive activities. In the placebo group both of these indices worsened.

Discussion

Aromatherapy with essential balm oil was well tolerated and performed statistically better than the placebo treatment. Restlessness and shouting were the domains with the greatest improvement and the quality of life indices also indicated a benefit in overall wellbeing for those in the active treatment group. The people in the placebo group also experienced an improvement in their agitation scores and this modest placebo effect could be explained by the increased social contact in both groups.

(Source: adapted from Lee et al., 2003)

Comment

1   There are often problems associated with attempts to ensure that the people administering a therapy are unaware whether it is the active treatment or the placebo. Obviously problems arise, for example, when investigating acupuncture or other forms of 'hands-on' therapies, because the people giving the therapy know what treatment has been involved. In this case the active aromatherapy ingredient is melissa (lemon balm) and attempts were made to ensure it was administered in exactly the same way as the non-active ingredient (sunflower oil) that was used as a placebo. However, these two ingredients smell and probably feel different, so the people administering the products could have been aware which was the 'active' substance being tested.

2   A person's capacity to give informed consent is a crucial issue in the care of people with dementia. A clinical trial such as this is no different from other treatments or interventions involving choice and informed consent (Wiles and Booker, 2005). Shah and Dickenson (1999) suggest that capacity to consent should be judged in relation to specific decisions, such as participating or not in a research trial. Agreement may be sufficient where there is a lack of full capacity to consent. Where a person clearly is unable to make an informed judgement, Fellows (1998) suggests that their prior preferences should be determined and that willing participation and apparent enjoyment could be interpreted as assent. In this research trial the issue of consent is complex and withholding potentially beneficial treatment when doing research to establish the efficacy of a simple form of treatment may have its own ethical problems.

Case Study 2: Does acupuncture help people with chronic headache?

This case study is based on a large-scale, pragmatic, randomised trial which studied various health-related outcomes in people with a particular symptom (headache) using a specific CAM therapy (acupuncture). The research effort in this project was necessarily greater in order to complete such a large-scale trial. Over 400 people were the subjects of the research and several researchers, therapists and primary care teams also became involved. In a trial like this people with certain symptoms are allocated randomly to two groups and the groups are then compared in terms of measurable response to treatment. This trial is called 'pragmatic', which implies that the treatment conditions are deliberately kept as close as possible to how they would be delivered in day-to-day practice. In this way it might be possible to allow for

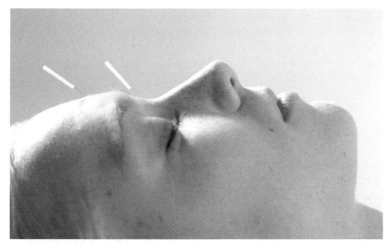

Can acupuncture alleviate chronic headache?

individual variations in the treatment given – say in the exact positions where the acupuncturist inserts the needles – rather than standardising a single approach (Thomas and Fitter, 2002).

ACTIVITY   USING ACUPUNCTURE FOR TREATING CHRONIC HEADACHE IN PRIMARY CARE

Allow 30 minutes

Read the description in Box 8.2 of research done by Andrew Vickers and his colleagues in England and Wales (Vickers et al., 2004). As you read, make notes in answer to the following questions.

1   What do you consider are the major strengths of this research?

2   What limitations do you think might be associated with the research?

BOX 8.2   ACUPUNCTURE FOR TREATING CHRONIC HEADACHE

Introduction

Vickers et al. (2004) report on a randomised controlled trial to determine the effects of a policy of 'use acupuncture' on headache, health status, days off sick, and use of resources in people with chronic headache compared with a policy of 'avoid acupuncture'. A total of 401 people were chosen from primary care settings who had chronic headaches, predominantly migraine. They were randomly allocated to receive up to 12 acupuncture treatments over three months or to a control intervention offering 'usual care'.

Migraine and tension-type headache give rise to notable health, economic and social costs. Despite the undoubted benefits of medication, many people continue to experience distress and social disruption. This leads people to try, and health professionals to recommend, non-pharmacological approaches to headache care. One of the most popular approaches seems to be acupuncture.

Accrual of participants

People's conditions were diagnosed as migraine or tension-type headache, following criteria of the International Headache Society (1988). People aged 18 to 65 who reported an average of at least two headaches per month were eligible. They completed a baseline headache diary for four weeks. Those who provided written informed consent, had a mean weekly baseline headache score of 8.75 or more, and completed at least 75 per cent of the baseline diary were randomised to a policy of 'use acupuncture' or 'avoid acupuncture'.

Treatment

People randomised to acupuncture received, in addition to standard care from general practitioners, up to 12 treatments over three months from an advanced member of the Acupuncture Association of Chartered Physiotherapists. The acupuncture point prescriptions used were individualised to each person and were at the discretion of the acupuncturist. People randomised to 'avoid acupuncture' received usual care from their general practitioner but were not referred to acupuncture.

Outcome assessment

People completed a daily diary of headache and medication use for four weeks at baseline and then three months and one year after randomisation. Severity of headache was recorded four times a day on a six-point Likert scale and the total summed to give a headache score. The SF-36 health status questionnaire was completed at baseline, three months, and one year. Every three months after randomisation, people completed additional questionnaires that monitored use of headache treatments and days sick from work or other usual activity. People were also contacted one year after randomisation and asked to give a global estimate of current and baseline headache severity on a 0 to 10 scale.

Results

In the primary analysis mean headache scores were significantly lower in the acupuncture group. Scores fell by 34 per cent in the acupuncture group compared with 16 per cent in controls. The difference in days with headache of 1.8 days per four weeks is equivalent to 22 fewer days of headache per year (8 to 38). The effects of acupuncture seem to be long lasting; although few people continued to receive acupuncture after the initial three-month treatment period, headache scores were lower at 12 months than at the follow up after treatment. Medication scores at follow up were lower in the acupuncture group, although differences between groups did not reach significance for all end points. Use of medication fell by 23 per cent in controls but by 37 per cent in the acupuncture group. SF-36 data generally favoured acupuncture, although differences reached significance only for physical role functioning, energy, and change in health.

> People in the acupuncture group made fewer visits to general practitioners and complementary practitioners than those not receiving acupuncture and took fewer days off sick. Confirming the excellent safety profile of acupuncture, the only adverse event reported was five cases of headache after treatment in four subjects.
>
> (Source: adapted from Vickers et al., 2004)

Comment

1   The methodological strengths of this study include a large sample size, concealed randomisation, and careful follow-up. The practical value of the trial was maximised by comparing the effects of clinically relevant alternatives on a diverse group of people recruited directly from primary care. The 'pragmatic' design of the trial ensures that the treatment given to the people receiving acupuncture is as close as possible to the acupuncturists' usual practice. However, it is not entirely clear which element of the treatment was responsible for the positive outcome of the trial: what can be claimed is that, in the context of current primary care organisations, a similar client population receiving a similar 'package' of care is likely to have a better outcome than those receiving standard care from general practitioners.

2   Control patients did not receive a sham acupuncture intervention. One hypothesis might be that the effects seen in the acupuncture group resulted not from the physiological action of needle insertion but from the 'placebo effect'. People in the trial obviously knew which arm of the research they were in (acupuncture or no acupuncture) and may therefore have given biased assessments of their headache scores. Patients recorded all treatments for headache during the course of the study. The use of medication and other therapies (such as chiropractic) was lower in patients assigned to acupuncture, indicating that the positive results in this group were not due to confounding by interventions outside the study.

Case Study 3: Does t'ai chi help people with fibromyalgia?

In this case study of CAM-related research, Helen Taggart and her colleagues set out to answer the specific question: 'Does t'ai chi exercise help people with fibromyalgia?' (Taggart et al., 2003). This research project focused on a group of people with a particular condition (fibromyalgia) and followed their progress when they used one specific type of CAM intervention (t'ai chi exercise). The research did not attempt to compare this group's experience of using t'ai chi with any other (control) group of people. This type of research is comparatively common because it is a straightforward inquiry that is accessible to many practitioners, and to researchers who do not have enormous resources at their disposal. Complex research techniques are not necessary to conduct this type of inquiry and no control groups were

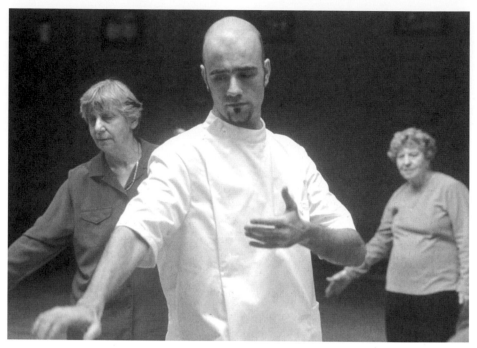

Can t'ai chi help people with fibromyalgia?

established for comparison with the active group. However, the conclusions that can be drawn from this type of research are also considerably limited. The research attempts to measure and understand the 'journey' of a group of people receiving a particular therapy.

ACTIVITY   RESEARCH WITHOUT A CONTROL GROUP

Allow 20 minutes

Read the report in Box 8.3 of the study by Helen Taggart and her colleagues in the USA (Taggart et al., 2003). The details of the statistical analysis have not been reproduced so that you can concentrate on other features of the design and outcomes of the research. As you read the report of this research project, make notes in answer to the following questions.

1   What are the advantages of a research project that does not use a control group?

2   What possible limitations are there to this type of research?

3   What sort of control groups could have been used to compare with this form of treatment?

BOX 8.3   EFFECTS OF T'AI CHI EXERCISE ON FIBROMYALGIA SYMPTOMS AND HEALTH-RELATED QUALITY OF LIFE

Background

■ Fibromyalgia (FM) is a common musculoskeletal disorder associated with multiple problems of pain in the limbs and inadequate or limited symptom relief. The cause of this complex syndrome is unknown, and there is no known cure. Although FM is one of the most common musculoskeletal disorders, its biophysical mechanisms are poorly understood. Impaired global health, high disability levels, decreased functional levels, and inadequate or limited symptom relief are common problems (Barnard et al., 2000; Paulson et al., 2002; Wassern et al., 2002).

■ T'ai chi is an ancient Chinese martial art form. The specific form used for this study is the Yang-style short form (Dunn, 1999). The intervention consisted of 1-hour, twice-weekly t'ai chi classes for six weeks.

Research hypotheses

■ The purpose of this study was to examine the benefits of t'ai chi exercise as an intervention to reduce FM symptoms and enhance health for individuals with FM. The hypotheses were that there would be (1) positive changes in pre-exercise to post-exercise scores for FM symptoms and (2) positive changes in pre-exercise to post-exercise scores for health status after six weeks of twice-weekly, 1-hour t'ai chi exercise classes.

Methods

■ Participants were recruited from a local Fibromyalgia Support Group. Inclusion criteria were: (1) self-reported diagnosis of FM; (2) ability to speak and understand English; (3) ability to ambulate independently; and (4) not currently enrolled in t'ai chi classes. Exclusion criteria were: (1) physician instructions to avoid physical activity; and (2) other rheumatic diseases or psychiatric disorders. Written informed consent was obtained from all participants included in the study. Baseline data collection before t'ai chi exercise included the Fibromyalgia Impact Questionnaire (FIQ) and the Medical Outcomes Study Questionnaire Short Form-36 (SF-36).

■ Participants then engaged in six weeks of twice-weekly, 1-hour t'ai chi classes. Post-exercise data collection included the FIQ and SF-36.

Fibromyalgia Impact Questionnaire

■ The FIQ (Burckhardt et al., 1991) is a 10-item, self-administered instrument that measures the impact of FM symptoms on physical functioning, ability to work, depression, anxiety, sleep, pain, stiffness, fatigue, morning tiredness, and well-being. This instrument has established reliability and validity and is sensitive to change (Bennett et al., 1996).

Short Form-36

■ The 36-item short form of the Medical Outcomes Study Questionnaire (SF-36) was designed as a generic indicator of health-related quality of life (Ware and Sherbourne, 1992). The SF-36 contains multi-item scales to measure eight dimensions: physical functioning, role limitations (physical), bodily pain, social functioning, general health, role limitations (emotional), vitality, and general health perceptions. Reliability and validity are well established (McDowell and Newell, 1996).

Description of the people sampled

■ Thirty-seven adults with FM volunteered to participate in the six-week t'ai chi classes. The sample was predominantly female (35 of 37). Of the 37 enrolled participants, two withdrew for family reasons, two could not do the exercises, one had back surgery, and nine had incomplete data sheets. After the period of research, ten of the participants continued the classes at their own expense, and an additional five participants reported that they do the exercises at home.

Results

■ **Changes in fibromyalgia symptoms** The results revealed statistically significant improvement in six FIQ domains: physical function, feeling good, pain, morning tiredness, stiffness and anxiety. Four domains — work missed, job ability, fatigue, and depression — did not reach statistical significance but showed positive clinical improvement.

■ **Changes in health-related quality of life** Physical functioning, bodily pain, general health, vitality, and emotional health revealed statistically significant improvement. The two domains physical and social functioning showed clinically significant improvement but did not reach statistical significance. The mental health domain showed the least improvement.

Additional findings

■ Participants volunteered comments regarding benefits of the t'ai chi exercise participation. One participant stated, 'I thoroughly enjoyed the classes of t'ai chi and thought it was very beneficial. I try to do some of the exercises each morning and find that it helps my neck and back.' Another participant stated, 'I participated in all 12 sessions and am planning to continue the t'ai chi program. My pain and stiffness are much less. I have more mental clarity and generally feel better. My breathing is better.'

Discussion

■ Data from this study support improvements in FM symptom management and health status for the participants in this study. The improved symptom management is similar to studies using drugs (Wolfe et al., 1995), pool exercises (Mannerkorpi et al., 2000), and qi gong, a Chinese movement therapy, combined with intensive education and relaxation therapy (Creamer et al., 2000).

■   The lack of statistically significant improvement in some domains might
    result from the short duration of the study or limitations in the FIQ
    research tool in assessing fatigue. Like the changes in scores for FM
    symptom management, changes in mean scores for the health status,
    using the SF-36, indicated pre- to post-t'ai chi improvement in each of
    the eight domains. This finding is similar to other exercise intervention
    studies (Mannerkorpi et al., 2000; Meyer and Lemley, 2000; Wigers et al.,
    1996). Lack of statistical significance in some domains may have resulted
    from the small number of participants and from the short duration of
    the study.

(Source: adapted from Taggart et al., 2003)

Comment

1   It is comparatively straightforward to organise this type of research. Although
    descriptive research sets out to answer a natural question, without comparison
    with other matched groups of people experiencing other forms of treatment
    (or even no treatment), ultimately the conclusions that can be drawn are
    rather limited. However, the advantage of a research project that does not use
    a control group is that it is comparatively simple to organise. The researchers
    took a group of 37 people and studied and measured their progress. This
    research can be done in one clinic, or, as in this research project, by recruiting
    people with the condition from a local, disease-specific support group.

2   A limitation of this study was the small sample size and the high number of
    participants not completing the study. Three participants withdrew for family
    or health reasons; two participants withdrew because they could not do the
    exercises. Also, the participants may want to 'please' the investigator; the
    time and effort invested by the participants may also influence their desire to
    report a positive outcome; and, of course, they were all recruited from one
    support group.

3   The symptoms of many diseases fluctuate and people get better or worse for a
    variety of reasons, so it is not possible to compare this 'treatment' group of
    people with another matched group of people with fibromyalgia who had no
    treatment at all. Sometimes, people feel better with the passage of time.
    Alternatively, it may have been possible to compare this group of people with
    another matched selection of people having a different type of treatment,
    such as another form of CAM, or some types of more orthodox treatment, such
    as using painkillers or muscle relaxants.

Case Study 4: Can acupuncture positively affect the physiological markers of active Crohn's disease?

This case study is about research into the effect of a CAM therapy (acupuncture) on a specific disease (Crohn's disease) using a physiologically measured outcome – in this case, serum markers of inflammation (α_1-acid glycoprotein and C-reactive protein):

> The use of a primary objective outcome (eg, urine toxicity screens in addiction studies) may protect against patient bias as well as staff bias influencing primary outcomes.
>
> (Margolin et al., 1998, p. 1627)

In the other research reports considered so far in this chapter, the outcome measures were based on whether the people in the studies felt better or worse after having some form of CAM intervention. It is argued that these sorts of outcomes introduce the possibility of bias into the research. In an attempt to eliminate such bias some research tries to use laboratory findings to quantify the effectiveness or otherwise of CAM interventions. The research question then is: 'Does the use of CAM lead to biochemical changes in the body?' In terms of the scientific method, this should provide a more objective measure of the treatment's effects.

ACTIVITY   USING PHYSIOLOGICAL MEASUREMENTS AS AN OUTCOME MEASURE

Allow 30 minutes

Read the description in Box 8.4 of research done in Germany by Stefanie Joos and her colleagues (Joos et al., 2004). As you read, make notes in answer to the following question.

■   Do you think it is important to measure physiological as well as observational features of disease progression when researching CAM interventions?

BOX 8.4   ACUPUNCTURE IN THE TREATMENT OF ACTIVE CROHN'S DISEASE: A RANDOMISED CONTROLLED STUDY

Background

Acupuncture has traditionally been used in the treatment of inflammatory bowel disease in China and is increasingly being applied in Western countries. The purpose of this study was to investigate the efficacy of acupuncture in the treatment of active Crohn's disease (CD).

Methods

A prospective, randomized, controlled, single-blind clinical trial was carried out to analyze the change in the CD activity index (CDAI) after treatment as a main outcome measure, and the changes in quality of life and general well-being and serum markers of inflammation (α_1-acid glycoprotein, C-reactive protein) as secondary outcome measures. 51 patients with mild to moderately active CD were treated in a single center for complementary medicine by three trained acupuncturists and randomly assigned to receive either traditional acupuncture (TCM group, n = 27) or control treatment at non-acupuncture points (control group, n = 24). Patients were treated in 10 sessions over a period of 4 weeks and followed up for 12 weeks.

Results

In the TCM group the CDAI decreased from 250 ± 51 to 163 ± 56 points as compared with a mean decrease from 220 ± 42 to 181 ± 46 points in the control group ... In both groups these changes were associated with improvements in general well-being and quality of life. With regard to general well-being, traditional acupuncture was superior to control treatment ... α_1-acid glycoprotein concentration fell significantly only in the TCM group.

Conclusions

Apart from a marked placebo effect, traditional acupuncture offers an additional therapeutic benefit in patients with mild to moderately active CD.

(Source: Joos et al., 2004, p. 131)

Comment

Specific physiological measurement of this sort is not always possible. Many disease processes cannot be measured in this way and do not have marker blood tests to assess disease progression. However, when this type of increasingly objective testing is available, it is possible to eliminate certain areas of bias from the research process. Research findings or outcomes are considered in biomedicine to be more robust if they have been determined in this way.

8.3   Systematic reviews of quantitative studies

How can any conclusions be drawn from the usually small clinical trials that are carried out in both the orthodox and, particularly, the CAM fields? One approach to the problem is to use a technique called **systematic review**, where the results of several small studies of a particular topic are collected together. These results are then pooled for the purpose of analysis, called **meta-analysis**. There are both advantages and drawbacks to such an approach. Obviously, the main advantage is that numbers of samples can be 'bumped up', making the subsequent statistical analysis more robust. However, this can mask a multitude of sins, particularly if the primary studies were flawed. The results of unreliable studies do not become more reliable by lumping them together, and it is generally accepted that less rigorous trials tend to yield more positive results (Linde, 2002).

Of course, it is important to ensure that all the studies in the systematic review asked the same experimental question, even if they did not use exactly the same methodology to obtain an answer. It can be very difficult to select the studies to include and, before starting the systematic review, the reviewer should make explicit the criteria that are used to include or exclude particular studies. For example, one criterion might be 'no study with sample numbers lower than 10 will be included'. If the methodology of the selected studies is varied, enough detail should be given to allow the reader to understand the range of conditions being tested. If the studies use significantly different methodologies, they should not be included in the same review. Finally, the systematic review itself should be justifiable: will the meta-analyses yield results that are clinically useful?

There are several other hazards when selecting data for inclusion in a systematic review, in particular, **publication bias**. This occurs when studies with undesired results (mostly negative) are less often published than those with desired results (mostly positive). Small negative or inconclusive studies are especially likely to be rejected for publication. Publication bias typically leads to overoptimistic results and conclusions in systematic reviews (Linde, 2002).

Therefore, there is a considerable onus on the reviewer to make sure that the studies included in a meta-analysis are truly representative of **all** the data pertinent to the topic, including unpublished material, where this can be found. The criteria for including studies for analysis must be clearly stated and due attention should be paid to excluding any seriously flawed studies. According to Linde (2002, p. 196), the criteria that should be used in the systematic reviewing process are as follows.

1   Is there a clearly defined experimental question?

2   Is the literature search comprehensive and does it avoid publication bias?

3   Are the inclusion and exclusion criteria clear and adequate?

4   Are the methods used described in appropriate detail?

5   Are the primary studies sufficiently similar to be comparable?

6   Are the findings relevant to clinical practice?

The Cochrane Collaboration (2004) is an international, non-profit, independent organisation, which advises on and oversees many systematic reviews of CAM. There is now a significant and reliable body of evidence about the safety and efficacy of many treatments, including CAM, based on carefully conducted meta-analyses.

The basic idea of meta-analysis is that larger sample numbers lead to more accurate statistics. However, because of the sort of test that must be applied to such varied data, the final statistic is often not P (the probability that any differences arose by chance) but another kind of measure. One that is often used is the **relative risk** factor. This is defined as the proportion of patients with an event in the experimental group, compared with the proportion of patients with the same event in the control group. An 'event' is any outcome defined in the study: for a test of efficacy it could be a cure; for a test of safety it could be a death.

It is generally accepted that conclusions drawn from a meta-analysis are more robust than those derived from smaller studies. However, this does not necessarily mean that meta-analyses can give easy answers to any clinical problem.

Case Study 5: A systematic review of herbal medicines for treating osteoarthritis

Many herbal medicines are used to treat osteoarthritis. This systematic review brings together 12 trials and two systematic reviews which have tested a range of different herbal medicines to determine their efficacy in treating osteoarthritis.

ACTIVITY   ARE HERBAL MEDICINES EFFECTIVE FOR TREATING OSTEOARTHRITIS?

Allow 30 minutes

Read the report of a systematic review by Long et al. (2001) in Box 8.5. As you read, check this systematic review against the following criteria.

■ Is there a clearly defined experimental question?

■ Is the literature search comprehensive and does it avoid publication bias?

■ Are the inclusion and exclusion criteria clear and adequate?

■ Are the findings relevant to clinical practice?

BOX 8.5   HERBAL MEDICINES FOR THE TREATMENT OF OSTEOARTHRITIS

Objective

Limitations in the conventional medical management of osteoarthritis indicate a real need for safe and effective treatment of osteoarthritis patients. Herbal medicines may provide a solution to this problem. The aim of this research was to review systematically all randomised controlled trials on the effectiveness of herbal medicines in the treatment of osteoarthritis and to answer the question: 'In patients with osteoarthritis, are herbal medicines and plant extracts effective and safe?'

Methods

Computerised literature searches were carried out on five electronic databases. Trial data were extracted in a standardised, predefined manner and assessed independently. Studies were selected if they were randomised controlled trials comparing one herbal treatment with a placebo or another active drug in patients with osteoarthritis. Studies focusing on back pain, osteoarthritic conditions of the spine, or on parenterally applied herbal preparations were excluded, as were studies that lacked essential methodological detail such as dosage, baseline data, and clinical end points.

Results

Twelve trials and two systematic reviews fulfilled the inclusion criteria. The authors found promising evidence for the effective use of some herbal preparations in the treatment of osteoarthritis. In addition, evidence suggesting that some herbal preparations reduce consumption of non-steroidal anti-inflammatory drugs was found. The reviewed herbal medicines appear relatively safe. Twelve trials and two systematic reviews met the selection criteria. One crossover trial comparing **Articulin-F** (an Ayurvedic herbomineral formulation) with placebo found that active treatment reduced severity of pain and disability score. Two trials compared **avocado/soybean unsaponifiables** with placebo and found that active treatment led to reduced non-steroidal anti-inflammatory drug consumption and improvement in the functional index and pain (one trial). A meta-analysis combining data from three trials found that **capsaicin cream** was better than placebo in reducing pain. One other trial comparing capsaicin cream with placebo found that active treatment reduced pain severity and tenderness on passive range of motion and physician palpation. Two trials compared **Devil's claw** with placebo and found a decrease in pain severity (two trials) and an increase in mobility (one trial) with active treatment. One trial compared **Eazmov** with **diclofenac** and found that Eazmov was inferior to diclofenac for both pain severity and disability score. One crossover trial compared **ginger extract** with ibuprofen or placebo and found that ibuprofen was more effective than both ginger extract and placebo. One trial compared **gitadyl** with ibuprofen and found no difference between the treatment groups. One systematic review of six trials evaluating the effectiveness of **phytodolor** found that this herbal formulation led to reduced pain, increased mobility, and reduced anti-inflammatory drug consumption. One trial compared **Reumalex** with placebo and found that active treatment led to a reduction in pain compared with placebo. One trial compared **nettle sting** with placebo and found that placebo led to greater reductions in both pain and disability. **Willow bark** (one trial) also led to a reduction in pain compared with placebo. The incidence of adverse effects for these herbal medicines was low.

Conclusion

In patients with osteoarthritis, some herbal medicines and plant extracts reduced pain and disability and improved mobility, with a low incidence of adverse effects.

(Source: adapted from Long et al., 2001, p. 779; Ribeiro, 2002, p. 57)

Comment

This research was established to respond to a clearly defined experimental question: 'Can a systematic review be used to establish the effectiveness of herbal medicines for the treatment of people with osteoarthritis?'

Although Box 8.5 is a heavily edited extract of the research report, the literature search seems comprehensive and inclusion (and exclusion) criteria appear to be clear and adequate.

Clinical workers and people seeking advice about treating osteoarthritis would find this research relevant to clinical practice. Having read the research report, workers within the orthodox medical care system would feel more confident in suggesting to people with osteoarthritis that they might seek additional (complementary) help from a herbalist. Herbalists would probably have to follow up some of the research reports used in the systematic analysis in order to inform their more specialist practice.

Case Study 6: Does homeopathy work?

Some meta-analyses attempt to tackle all the available evidence that might answer a very general question, such as 'Does acupuncture work?' Linde et al. (2001) advise extreme caution when using reviews that claim to answer a question which has such a wide scope:

> This annotated bibliography of systematic reviews should also be interpreted with great caution. The risk of oversimplification in a systematic review is great. In a review of reviews it is extreme. We summarise the conclusion of a systematic review in a single phrase. Clinical decisions for treatment of individual patients should not be based on our work. For this, patients and health care professionals have to turn to the original reviews. Our aim was to provide a clear summary of what is available and where further information can be found. We tried to be as comprehensive as possible in our search but cannot exclude that we have overlooked eligible work, particularly if this was not published in a journal.
>
> (Linde et al., 2001, p. 10)

ACTIVITY   EVALUATION OF AN ENTIRE CAM THERAPY BY OVERVIEWING SYSTEMATIC REVIEWS

Allow 30 minutes

Read Box 8.6 (overleaf) which is about an overview of the research evidence on the effectiveness of one of the most established CAM modalities — homeopathy (O'Meara et al., 2002).

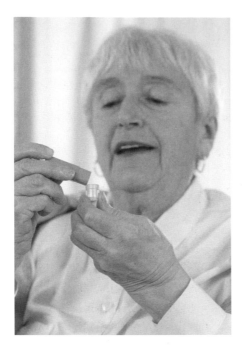

Does homeopathy work?

As you read, make notes in answer to the following questions.

■ How have the authors attempted to determine the effectiveness of the entire CAM modality of homeopathy?

■ What problems do you think might arise when attempting to consider such a wide question?

BOX 8.6   THE EFFECTIVENESS OF HOMEOPATHY

Summarising the research evidence

For this review, literature searches were initially done to identify systematic reviews of homeopathy. The Cochrane Library and the DARE database were searched. Reviews were assessed according to the following criteria: selection criteria for primary studies; literature search; validity assessment of primary studies; presentation of details of individual primary studies; and data summary.

Titles and abstracts were examined for relevance by two independent reviewers. Full papers were examined by two reviewers. Data were extracted and methodological quality was assessed by one reviewer and checked by a second reviewer. All disagreements were resolved by discussion.

Nature of the evidence

Around 200 randomised controlled trials (RCTs) evaluating homeopathy have been conducted, and there are also several systematic reviews of these trials. This review is based mainly on an overview of existing systematic reviews of RCTs.

Most RCTs of homeopathy have involved small numbers of patients and have suffered from low statistical power.

Reviews with a general scope

Four systematic reviews were identified. The purpose of these reviews was to determine whether there is any evidence for the effectiveness of homeopathic treatment generally. Patients with any disease were included, as opposed to investigating effects within a specific group, for example people with asthma. All reviews identified methodological problems with the primary studies and, as such, were unable to draw firm conclusions about the general effectiveness of homeopathy.

Reviews of individualised (classical) homeopathy

In classical or individualised homeopathy, practitioners aim to identify a single homeopathic preparation that matches a patient's general 'constitution'. Due to differences in elements of patients' constitutions, two patients with identical conventional diagnoses may receive different homeopathic prescriptions.

Two reviews were identified. Again, the scope of these reviews was general and selection criteria relating to participant characteristics and outcome measurements were unspecified. Methodological problems with the primary studies were reported in both reviews.

Reviews with a more specific scope

Eight reviews were identified with a specific focus in terms of the homeopathic agent being evaluated or the type of participants recruited.

Arnica

One review focused on the effectiveness of homeopathic arnica. Findings did not indicate that homeopathic arnica is any more effective than placebo. Some study details were lacking, particularly with regard to results and methodological quality, and therefore it is difficult to assess the reliability of the evidence.

Post-operative ileus (bowel muscle paralysis)

One review assessed the effectiveness of homeopathic treatment versus placebo in resolving post-operative ileus, and included six trials (four were RCTs) of patients undergoing abdominal or gynaecological surgery. Findings indicated that homeopathic treatment administered immediately after abdominal surgery may reduce recovery time when compared with placebo. However, the possibility of bias and inappropriate pooling of data means that these findings should be treated with caution. In addition, the largest and most well-conducted study, as rated by the authors of the review, showed no difference between homeopathy and placebo.

Delayed-onset muscle soreness (DOMS)

The effectiveness of homeopathy in reducing DOMS was assessed in a review of eight trials, including three RCTs. The results suggested that homeopathic remedies were no more effective than placebo in alleviating DOMS. The three RCTs all reported non-significant differences between treatment groups, while results from the non-randomised studies were inconsistent.

Arthritis and other musculoskeletal disorders

Two reviews were identified. One examined the effectiveness of homeopathy in people with rheumatoid arthritis, osteoarthritis, and other types of musculoskeletal disorders. The review included six placebo-controlled RCTs. Most of the trials were rated by the review's authors as being of high methodological quality. Although the overall pooled estimate indicated that homeopathy was superior to placebo, the data were clinically heterogeneous. In addition, the outcome measurements used in the pooling were not defined, but, when referring to a related publication, it seems likely that these were highly heterogeneous. Therefore, the findings of this review should be treated with caution.

The second review focused more specifically on osteoarthritis and included four RCTs. Fixed, rather than individualised, treatments were used in all trials. Results between trials were inconsistent and the authors noted methodological problems in all trials. This meant that firm conclusions could not be drawn.

Headaches/migraine

One systematic review focused on the effectiveness of homeopathy as a prophylactic agent for headaches and migraine. Results suggested that homeopathy was not effective. Four trials of classical homeopathy versus placebo were included. One trial of poor methodological quality found a statistically significant improvement in all outcomes in favour of homeopathy, whereas the trials of better quality all reported no statistically significant differences between groups.

Asthma

A well-conducted review assessed the effectiveness of homeopathy in treating stable chronic asthma or asthma-like symptoms. The three included RCTs were of variable methodological quality. Two showed results in favour of homeopathy (symptom improvement, lung function improvement, and less use of corticosteroids) and one found no statistically significant differences between groups.

Influenza

A good quality systematic review assessed the use of homeopathic oscillococcinum in preventing and treating influenza. Problems with methodological quality and reporting were noted in all the trials. No further RCTs were identified concerning the use of homeopathic oscillococcinum, or any other homeopathic preparation, in preventing or treating influenza.

Induction of labour

One systematic review assessing the role of homeopathy for the induction of labour was identified. Only one RCT (n = 40) was identified, which compared homeopathic caulophyllum with placebo. Although statistically significant differences were found between treatment groups, this trial may have been too small to detect the true treatment effect.

Implications

The evidence base for homeopathy needs to be interpreted with caution. Many of the areas that have been researched are not representative of the conditions that homeopathic practitioners usually treat. Additionally, all conclusions about effectiveness should be considered together with the methodological inadequacies of the primary studies and some of the systematic reviews.

There are currently insufficient data either to recommend homeopathy as a treatment for any specific condition, or to warrant significant changes in the provision of homeopathy.

(Source: adapted from O'Meara et al., 2002)

Comment

There are several problems and controversies surrounding the existing evidence base for homeopathy. First, there is much debate about whether homeopathy shows any effect over and above placebo (the dummy medication or treatment given to participants in trials). Sceptics have argued that homeopathy cannot work because remedies are diluted to such a degree that not even a single molecule of the active substance remains. Given the absence of a plausible mechanism of action, they argue that the existing evidence base represents little more than a series of placebo versus placebo trials:

> How seriously clinicians take these findings [about the effectiveness of homeopathy] depends on their prior beliefs. If you cannot conceive of highly diluted solutions with undetectable drug concentrations having a positive effect, then no matter how well designed the trial, or robust the meta-analysis, a positive result will not change your view.
>
> (Feder and Katz, 2002, p. 499)

Advocates have argued that much of the research into the effectiveness of homeopathy is not representative of routine homeopathic practice because homeopathic treatment is highly individualised: that is, two patients showing similar symptoms may receive different treatments. While it is possible to carry out RCTs of the efficacy of homeopathy, researchers have tended to focus on conducting placebo-controlled RCTs, either to test the effects of a single remedy on a particular condition and/or to explore the placebo issue. So, conditions such as delayed-onset muscle soreness have been studied whereas skin conditions such as eczema, which homeopaths commonly treat, have been overlooked.

Unease with the usefulness of this type of research into homeopathy and other holistic CAM therapies has led many researchers to advocate the use of qualitative methods.

8.4   Adding qualitative methods

A major dilemma in CAM is whether it can be justified within a biomedical paradigm, using the scientific method to prove its efficacy, or whether a case should be made for operating within a different, more holistic paradigm, where qualitative and possibly longitudinal methods are more appropriate:

> Qualitative research can assist in understanding the meaning of an intervention to patients as well as patients' beliefs about the treatment and expectations of the outcome. Qualitative research also assists in understanding the impact of the context and the process of the intervention. Finally, qualitative research is helpful in developing appropriate outcome measures for CAM interventions.
>
> (Verhoef et al., 2002, p. 275)

These arguments were discussed in Chapter 7. This section describes some attempts to use qualitative methods to investigate CAM use.

Case Study 7: Using qualitative methods to investigate (a) acupuncture and (b) qi gong for people with muscular dystrophy

This case study summarises two qualitative research studies which used **grounded theory**. This method was originally developed by Glaser and Strauss (1967) to study dying patients' awareness of their situation. It has been used extensively in nursing research. It is a method of generating theory rather than testing theory. So, unlike most research within the scientific method tradition, which aims to test hypotheses, grounded theory generates hypotheses. The data gathered from face-to-face interviews, observation from field notes and other data-collection techniques used in qualitative research are analysed in a particular way. In most traditional research the analysis does not begin until all the data are collected: that is, only after all the experiments have finished or all the questionnaires are completed. In grounded theory research the analysis starts soon after data collection begins, typically at the time of the first interviews. In fact, one of the strengths of the grounded theory approach is that the ongoing analysis can inform the way the data are collected. Sheila Payne describes the main stages in grounded theory analysis as follows.

1   Development of categories to describe the data: Close examination of the transcripts are used to identify categories which describe the data. These categories closely fit the data and are not imposed by previous theories.

2   Saturation of categories: The initial selection of categories is dependent upon the first interviews analyzed. However, as additional examples of the phenomenon are discovered in subsequent transcripts, the categories become saturated. The discovery of new categories in later analyses may necessitate re-analysis of previously processed transcripts.

3   Definition of categories: As sufficient instances of a particular category are developed, it is possible to define it. The definition is used to place limits and boundaries around a category, enabling it to be compared and contrasted with other categories. After definition, categories are integrated to form a grounded theory. To achieve integration, it is necessary to formulate a storyline around the central phenomenon of the study. This involves relating the central phenomenon or 'core category' to other categories. The categories are arranged and re-arranged until they seem to fit the story, and provide an analytical version.

(Payne, 1997, p. 106)

Attempts are usually made to link the grounded theories generated in this way to other existing theories, to add to or question the body of knowledge on the topic under consideration. However, the theory must also be tested, perhaps by revisiting the data or by interviewing the participants again so they can comment on the emerging theory (Payne, 1997).

ACTIVITY   TWO STUDIES USING QUALITATIVE METHODS

Allow 30 minutes

Read the summaries of two research studies in Boxes 8.7 and 8.8. As you read, make notes on what these studies claim to achieve. What are the possible limitations of these types of study?

BOX 8.7   ACUPUNCTURE AS A COMPLEX INTERVENTION: A HOLISTIC MODEL

Objectives

Our understanding of acupuncture and Chinese medicine is limited by a lack of inquiry into the dynamics of the process. We used a longitudinal research design to investigate how the experience, and the effects, of a course of acupuncture evolved over time.

Design and outcome measures

This was a longitudinal qualitative study, using a constant comparative method, informed by grounded theory. Each person was interviewed three times over 6 months. Semi-structured interviews explored people's experiences of illness and treatment. Across-case and within-case analysis resulted in themes and individual vignettes.

Subjects and settings

Eight professional acupuncturists in seven different settings informed their patients about the study. We interviewed a consecutive sample of 23 people with chronic illness, who were having acupuncture for the first time.

Results

People described their experience of acupuncture in terms of the acupuncturist's diagnostic and needling skills; the therapeutic relationship; and a new understanding of the body and self as a whole being. All three of these components were imbued with holistic ideology. Treatment effects were perceived as changes in symptoms, changes in energy, and changes in personal and social identity. The vignettes showed the complexity and the individuality of the experience of acupuncture treatment. The process and outcome components were distinct but not divisible, because they were linked by complex connections.

Conclusions

The holistic model of acupuncture treatment, in which 'the whole being greater than the sum of the parts', has implications for service provision and for research trial design. Research trials that evaluate the needling technique, isolated from other aspects of process, will interfere with treatment outcomes.

(Source: abstract of Paterson and Britten, 2004)

BOX 8.8　A QUALITATIVE STUDY OF A NOVEL EXERCISE PROGRAMME FOR PATIENTS WITH MUSCULAR DYSTROPHY

Muscular dystrophy patients have often experimented with different alternative or complementary methods since there is at present no curative medical treatment.

Purpose

To evaluate, through qualitative analysis of interview data, the subjective experiences of twenty-eight patients with muscular dystrophy practising a complementary method, qi gong.

Methods

Semi-structured qualitative interviews were performed and data were analysed by a method inspired by Grounded Theory. The material was first coded into 119 categories, thereafter condensed to 59 categories through a constant comparison analysis. In the final analysis, six broad categories were formed out of these 59 categories.

Results

These broad categories were:

1   experience of health care and alternative methods
2   expectations, acceptance and compliance
3   qi gong as an adaptable form of exercise
4   stress reduction and mental effects
5   increased body awareness and physical effects
6   psychosocial effects of group training.

Conclusion

Qi gong was accepted as a novel exercise regimen and there was a wide variation of experience regarding it among the participants. Depending upon factors such as expectation of benefits, time available to do qi gong and perceived effects [of] doing it, compliance varied. One major advantage of qi gong is the ability to adapt the different exercises to the physical capability of the person practising qi gong. There were reports of mental, physical and psychosocial effects of the qi gong, which reduced the feeling of stress and improved well-being.

(Source: abstract of Wenneberg et al., 2004)

Comment

Neither of these studies attempted simply to test whether the therapies were effective. Instead, they tried to discover more about, as Paterson and Britten put it, **the dynamics of the process**. They showed the complexity and individuality of the experience of acupuncture. Wenneberg et al. identified a wide variation of experience of qi gong. These findings have important implications for practitioners in that they provide information on how people use and benefit from the therapies investigated. Of course, they are both based on very subjective views, which in qualitative research terms is a strength, but, in terms of the scientific method, which favours objective data, this is a limitation. Also in terms of the scientific method, the strength of providing insight into the complexity of individual experience is a limitation because it is hard to generalise from the findings.

The acupuncture study claims to have implications for the design of quantitative research trials. One of the most productive ways of doing research is to combine qualitative and quantitative methods. This is considered to be a way forward for CAM research.

8.5   Combining methods in CAM research

Chapter 7 argued that the scientific method and more qualitative methods reflect different world views, but there are many voices in CAM arguing that these methods are not incompatible and that, in fact, they can productively complement each other (Ribeaux and Spence, 2001; Verhoef et al., 2002):

> although RCTs have an important place in the assessment of the efficacy of CAM, the addition of qualitative research methods to RCTs can greatly enhance the understanding of CAM. Such additions have the potential to improve CAM interventions, and, thus, health care delivery.
>
> (Verhoef et al., 2002, p. 275)

In what ways can they combine and complement each other? The case studies in this section describe just two of a growing number of studies in the CAM field that combine qualitative and quantitative methods.

Case Study 8: Combining methods in a study of music therapy and cancer patients and a survey of users of Chinese medicine

The two research studies described here both used quantitative and qualitative methods but were very different in their scope and purpose. The first is a small-scale pilot study into the effects of music therapy on cancer

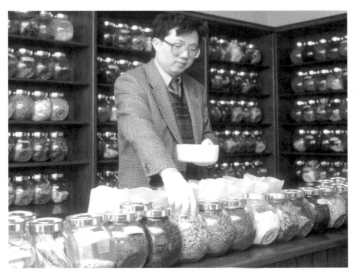

Users of Chinese medicine value their relationship with the practitioner

patients at the Bristol Cancer Help Centre, which combines quantitative, pre/post-test psychological and physiological measures with a qualitative focus group. The other is a large-scale sample survey of Chinese medicine users in the USA combined with handwritten stories of the respondents' experience of using Chinese medicines.

ACTIVITY   TWO ATTEMPTS AT COMBINING RESEARCH METHODS

Allow 45 minutes

Read the summaries of the two research studies in Boxes 8.9 and 8.10. In which ways do you think the qualitative and quantitative methods complement each other in these studies?

BOX 8.9   A PILOT STUDY OF THE THERAPEUTIC EFFECTS OF MUSIC THERAPY AT A CANCER HELP CENTRE

Context

Since the mid-1980s, music therapy has been a regular feature of the residential program at the internationally renowned Bristol Cancer Help Centre, United Kingdom. Music therapy complements other therapeutic interventions available to residents at the center.

Objective

To compare the therapeutic effects of listening to music in a relaxed state with the active involvement of music improvisation (the playing of tuned and untuned percussion instruments) in a music therapy group setting and to investigate the potential influence of music therapy on positive emotions and the immune system of cancer patients.

Design

A quantitative pre-posttest, psychological/physiological measures, and qualitative focus group design.

Setting

A cancer help center that offers a fully integrated range of complementary therapies, psychological support, spiritual healing, and nutritional and self-help techniques addressing the physical, mental, emotional, and spiritual needs of cancer patients and their supporters.

Participants

Twenty-nine cancer patients, aged 21 to 68 years.

Intervention

Group music therapy interventions of listening to recorded/live music in a relaxed state and improvisation.

Main outcome measures

Increased well-being and relaxation and less tension during the listening experience. Increased well-being and energy and less tension during improvisation. Increased levels of salivary immunoglobulin A and decreased levels of cortisol in both experiences.

Results

Psychological data showed increased well-being and relaxation as well as altered energy levels in both interventions. Physiological data showed increased salivary immunoglobulin A in the listening experience and a decrease in cortisol levels in both interventions over a 2-day period. Preliminary evidence of a link between positive emotions and the immune system of cancer patients was found.

(Source: Burns et al., 2001, p. 48)

BOX 8.10　CHINESE MEDICINE USERS IN THE USA

Part I: Utilisation, satisfaction and medical plurality

Objectives

Chinese medicine is growing in popularity and offers an important alternative or complement to biomedical care, but little is known of who uses it or why they purchase it. This article reports the first in-depth, large scale (n = 575) survey of United States acupuncture users.

Design

An anonymous mixed quantitative-qualitative survey questionnaire assessed user demographics, Chinese medicine modalities used, complaints, response to care, other health-care used, and satisfaction with care in six general-service clinics in five states.

Results and conclusions

The user demographic picture was of mid-age, well-educated, employed, mid-income patients. They sought care for a wide variety of conditions; top uses were for relief of musculoskeletal dysfunction, mood care, and wellness care. A large majority reported 'disappearance' or 'improvement' of symptoms, improved quality of life, and reduced use of selected measures including prescription drugs and surgery. Respondents reported utilizing a wide array of practices in addition to Chinese medicine, while also expressing extremely high satisfaction with Chinese medicine care. The evidence indicates that these respondents behave as astute customers within a plural health care system.

(Source: Cassidy, 1998a, p. 17)

Part II: Preferred aspects of care

Objectives

While a limited amount of data describe who seeks Chinese medicine care and for what conditions, there have been few attempts to explain what users think the care does for them, or why they value and 'like' the care. This article presents such data via an analysis of a sample of 460 handwritten stories collected as part of a mixed quantitative qualitative survey of 6 acupuncture clinics in 5 states.

Results

Quantitative data collected in this survey (Part I) showed that respondents were highly satisfied with their Chinese medicine care. The qualitative analysis found that respondents valued relief of presenting complaints as well as expanded effects of care including improvements in physiological and psychosocial adaptivity. In addition, respondents reported enjoying a close relationship with their Chinese medicine practitioner, learning new things, and feeling more able to guide their own lives and care for themselves. While these factors mesh well with Chinese medicine theory, respondents did not reveal familiarity with that theory. Instead, their language and experiences indicate familiarity with an holistic model of healthcare – and they seem to have experienced Chinese medicine care as holistic care.

Conclusions

This finding matters because it shows that respondents are not seeking an 'exotic' kind of healthcare, but are utilizing a homegrown, if non-mainstream, model of healthcare. The finding also matters because it shows that an holistic health delivery model is not only feasible, but currently exists in the United States: how Chinese medicine practitioners are trained, and how they subsequently deliver their care, could serve as a model for American healthcare reform.

(Source: Cassidy, 1998b, p. 189)

Comment

In the small-scale pilot study described in Box 8.9 the quantitative pre- and post-test data, which used psychological measurements of relaxation and altered energy levels and the physiological measurements of salivary immunoglobulin A and levels of cortisol, provided objective data of improved wellbeing. This was complemented by the subjective and more detailed account of the experience which came out of the qualitative data from the focus group.

In the large-scale survey of the use of Chinese medicine in the USA, the quantitative survey provided data which enabled the researchers to build up a picture of the type of people who used Chinese medicine, the conditions for which they used it and the benefits they derived from it. They also found high levels of satisfaction. The qualitative handwritten stories provided more details about the benefits and the satisfaction gained. For instance, the author found that the respondents valued the close relationship that they felt they had with their Chinese medicine practitioner, they learned new facts and they felt more in control of their own lives and care. The author also found that the respondents were interested less in the actual theoretical basis of Chinese medicine but valued it because it was holistic care.

The qualitative and quantitative findings within each of these two studies did not conflict but complemented each other, providing a fuller picture than would have been the case if only one methodology had been used. However, what if the two types of data produced conflicting findings? What if, say, the music therapy had shown no increase in the objective psychological and physiological data and yet the subjective qualitative data still indicated an increase in wellbeing? Would the qualitative data seem less convincing? If so, perhaps a larger-scale study would shed more light on the reasons why the respondents felt an improvement in their wellbeing and other psychological and physiological tests could be tried. Combining methodologies seems eminently sensible as a way forward for CAM research but it will not solve all the difficulties that have been identified in trying to research the diverse modalities that make up CAM.

8.6   Conclusion

This chapter took a critical look at some of the research methods used to study CAM by describing research of different degrees of complexity and asking a wide range of research questions. The problem of organising the necessary capacity to do CAM-related research was not tackled but it remains a problem. In the current climate, where most research activity is funded and dominated by drug companies and research workers who remain largely part of the orthodox establishment, it remains difficult to identify finance for CAM research. Perhaps this situation is beginning to change. For example, Feder and Katz consider that in relation to homeopathy:

> orthodox medicine has had the upper hand in terms of institutional support, research funding, and strong evidence of effectiveness. Nevertheless, the flurry of trials in the past 20 years has changed the terms of the debate. At the very least, those who consider homoeopathy to be absurd have had to muster different philosophical and methodological arguments to defend their position. Randomised controlled trials may be efficient arbiters of clinical effectiveness, but they are not particularly good for resolving philosophical disputes.
>
> (Feder and Katz, 2002, p. 498)

Some of the philosophical disputes seem to be as strong as ever. The research described earlier in this chapter takes a very firm orthodox scientific paradigm as its starting point. If CAM cannot be scrutinised in this way, how can it claim a place in the panoply of effective treatments that people might choose to help them remain healthy, or treat them when they are ill? However, people seem to choose treatment by CAM modalities, even those where there is no 'scientific' evidence base to back its claims. Lewith (2004, p. 4) believes this might be as much a problem for the researchers as for the users of CAM: 'there is little point in research denying what seems an apparent truth to an individual who has received effective acupuncture or homeopathy, as that only serves to undermine research by demonstrating its apparent ignorance.'

The world of CAM is divided between people who want to submit their therapies to the rigors of currently available 'scientific' testing and those who consider that CAM is based on such different principles from orthodox medicine that 'scientific' testing is inevitably futile. However, there is a growing interest in acknowledging that different methods can provide important data for CAM modalities and that combining methods is the way forward for a stronger research base for CAM.

KEY POINTS

- How seriously the results of specific CAM research should be taken can be determined by considering its 'provenance'. It is important to consider what sort of research it is, who did it and where it was published when assessing the value of any individual published research study.

- There is a growing, accumulated mass of evidence using the scientific method to determine the effectiveness of many different types of CAM intervention. Although there are no definitive answers to every question, the research effort in CAM is slowly giving meaningful results.

- Researching the effects of a CAM intervention on a group of people may reveal interesting results, but they are less convincing if no biomedical control group is used for comparison.

- Using a control group may be necessary within a biomedical paradigm but setting up a control group may not be feasible for many CAM therapies.

- Pragmatic trials are useful because the treatment given to respondents is similar to the treatment that people receive in a normal clinical setting.

- Systematic reviews of research findings add power to them but there are many significant pitfalls when ensuring that the results are valid.

- Even meta-analysis, which involves pooling all available systematic reviews, may not give answers to CAM-related research questions.

- Many CAM practitioners are unhappy about research done within the orthodox scientific method tradition, claiming it is reductionist and cannot possibly reveal the holistic effects of many CAM interventions.

- Drawing on a wide range of methods derived from the scientific method and from more qualitative methodologies is seen as a way forward for doing justice to the complex and holistic nature of CAM.

References

Anon. (1996) 'Integration of behavioural and relaxation approaches into the treatment of chronic pain and insomnia. NIH Technology Assessment Panel on Integration of Behavioural and Relaxation Approaches into the Treatment of Chronic Pain and Insomnia', *Journal of the American Medical Association*, Vol. 276, No. 4, pp. 313–8.

Ballard, C. G., O'Brien, J. T., Reichelt, K. and Perry, E. K. (2002) 'Aromatherapy as a safe and effective treatment for the management of agitation in severe dementia: the results of a double-blind, placebo controlled trial with *Melissa*', *Journal of Clinical Psychiatry*, Vol. 63, No. 7, pp. 553–8.

Barnard, A. L., Prince, A. and Edsall, P. (2000) 'Quality of life issues for fibromyalgia patients', *Arthritis Care and Research*, Vol. 13, No. 1, pp. 42–50.

Bennett, R., Burckhardt, C., Clark, S., O'Reilly, C., Wiens, A. and Campbell, S. (1996) 'Group treatment of fibromyalgia: a 6-month outpatient program', *Journal of Rheumatology*, Vol. 23, pp. 521–8.

Burckhardt, C., Clark, S. and Bennett, R. (1991) 'The fibromyalgia impact questionnaire: development and validation', *Journal of Rheumatology*, Vol. 18, No. 5, pp. 728–33.

Burns, A., Byrne, J., Ballard, C. and Holmes, C. (2002) 'Sensory stimulation in dementia: an effective option for managing behavioural problems', *British Medical Journal*, Vol. 325, pp. 1312–13.

Burns, S. J. I., Harbuz, M. S., Hucklebridge, F. and Bunt, L. (2001) 'A pilot study into the therapeutic effects of music therapy at a cancer help center', *Alternative Therapies in Health and Medicine*, Vol. 7, No. 1, pp. 48–56.

Cassidy, C. M. (1998a) 'Chinese medicine users in the United States. Part I: utilization, satisfaction, medical plurality', *The Journal of Alternative and Complementary Medicine*, Vol. 4, No. 1, pp 17–27.

Cassidy, C. M. (1998b) 'Chinese medicine users in the United States. Part II: preferred aspects of care', *The Journal of Alternative and Complementary Medicine*, Vol. 4, No. 2, pp. 189–202.

Cheung, N.-K. V., Modak, S., Vickers, A. and Knuckles, B. (2002) 'Orally administered β-glucans enhance anti-tumor effects of monoclonal antibodies', *Cancer Immunology and Immunotherapy*, Vol. 51, No. 10, pp. 557–64.

Cochrane Collaboration (2004) *A Brief Introduction*, London, Cochrane Collaboration. Available online at: www.cochrane.org/resources/leaflet.pdf [accessed 12 November 2004].

Creamer, P., Singh, B. B., Hochberg, M. C. and Berman, B. M. (2000) 'Sustained improvement produced by nonpharmacologic intervention in fibromyalgia: results of a pilot study', *Arthritis Care and Research*, Vol. 13, No. 4, pp. 198–204.

Di Blasi, Z. (2003) 'The crack in the biomedical box: the placebo effect', *The Psychologist*, Vol. 16, No. 2, pp. 72–5.

Dunn, T. (1999) *T'ai Chi for Health* [video], Venice, CA, Healing Arts.

Eisenberg, D., Davis, R., Ettner, S., Appel, S., Wilkey, S. and Van Rompay, M. (1998) 'Trends in alternative medicine use in the United States, 1990–1997: results of a follow-up national survey', *Journal of the American Medical Association*, Vol. 280, pp. 1569–75.

Ernst, E. (2002) 'What's the point of rigorous research on complementary/alternative medicine?', *Journal of the Royal Society of Medicine*, Vol. 95, pp. 211–13.

Feder, G. and Katz, T. (2002) Editorial: 'Randomised controlled trials for homoeopathy', *British Medical Journal*, Vol. 324, pp. 498–9.

Fellows, L. (1998) 'Competency and consent in dementia', *Journal of the American Geriatrics Society*, Vol. 46, pp. 922–6.

Filshie, J. and Cummings, T. (1999) 'Western medical acupuncture', in Ernst, E. and White, A. (eds) *Acupuncture: A Scientific Appraisal*, Oxford, Butterworth Heinemann.

Finkel, S., Burns, A. and Cohen, G. (2000) 'Behavioural and psychological symptoms of dementia: a clinical and research update', *International Psychogeriatrics*, Vol. 12 (s1), pp. 13–18.

Glaser, B. G. and Strauss, A. L. (1967) *The Discovery of Grounded Theory: Strategies for Qualitative Research*, New York, Aldine.

Grimm, R. (2002) 'Conducting multicenter and large trials in complementary and alternative medicine', in Lewith, G., Jonas, W. B. and Walach, H. (eds) *Clinical Research in Complementary Therapies*, pp. 139–53, Edinburgh, Churchill Livingstone.

International Headache Society (1988) 'Classification and diagnostic criteria for headache disorders, cranial neuralgias and facial pain', *Cephalagia*, Vol. 8, pp. 1–96.

Joos, S., Brinkhaus, B., Maluche, C., Maupai, N., Kohnen, R., Kraemer, N., Hahn, E. G. and Schuppan, D. (2004) 'Acupuncture and moxibustion in the treatment of active Crohn's disease: a randomized controlled study', *Digestion*, Vol. 69, pp. 131–9.

Kitwood, T. and Bredin, K. (1992) 'A new approach to the evaluation of dementia care', *Journal of Advances in Health and Nursing Care*, Vol. 1, No. 5, pp. 41–60.

Lee, L., Reichelt, K., Ballard, C. and Perry, E. (2003) 'Melissa aromatherapy as safe and effective treatment', *Nursing and Residential Care*, Vol. 5, No. 2, pp. 80–82.

Lewith, G. (2004) 'Can practitioners be researchers?', *Complementary Therapies in Medicine*, Vol. 12, pp. 2–5.

Linde, K. (2002) 'Systematic reviews and metaanalyses', in Lewith, G., Jonas, W. B. and Walach, H. (eds) *Clinical Research in Complementary Therapies*, pp. 187–97, Edinburgh, Churchill Livingstone.

Linde, K., Vickers, A., Hondras, M., ter Riet, G., Thormählen, J., Berman, B. and Melchart, D. (2001) 'Systematic reviews of complementary therapies – an annotated bibliography. Part 1: Acupuncture', *BMC Complementary and Alternative Medicine*, Vol. 1, No. 3, pp. 1–12.

Long, L., Soeken, K. and Ernst, E. (2001) 'Herbal medicines for the treatment of osteoarthritis: a systematic review', *Rheumatology*, Vol. 40, pp. 779–93.

Mannerkorpi, K., Nyberg, B., Ahlmen, M. and Ekdahl, C. (2000) 'Pool exercise combined with an education program for patients with fibromyalgia syndrome: a prospective, randomized study', *Journal of Rheumatology*, Vol. 27, pp. 2473–9.

Margolin, A., Avants, S. K. and Kleber, H. D. (1998) 'Investigating alternative medicine therapies in randomized controlled trials', *Journal of the American Medical Association*, Vol. 280, No. 18, pp. 1626–8.

McDowell, L. and Newell, C. (1996) *Measuring Health: A Guide to Rating Scales and Questionnaires* (2nd edition), New York, Oxford University.

Meade, T., Dyer, S., Browne, W., Townsend, J. and Frank, A. (1990) 'Low back pain of mechanical origin: randomised comparison of chiropractic and hospital outpatient treatment', *British Medical Journal*, Vol. 300, pp. 1431–7.

Meyer, B. B. and Lemley, K. H. (2000) 'Utilizing exercise to affect the symptomology of fibromyalgia: a pilot study', *Medicine and Science in Sports & Exercise*, Vol. 32, No. 10, pp. 1691–7.

O'Meara, S., Wilson, P., Bridle, C., Kleijnen, J. and Wright, K. (2002) 'Homeopathy', *Effective Health Care*, Vol. 7, No. 3, pp. 1–12.

Paterson, C. and Britten, N. (2004) 'Acupuncture as a complex intervention: a holistic model', *Journal of Alternative and Complementary Medicine*, Vol. 10, No. 5, pp. 791–801.

Paulson, M., Danielson, E. and Soderberg, S. (2002) 'Struggling for a tolerable existence: the meaning of men's lived experiences of living with pain of fibromyalgia type', *Qualitative Health Research*, Vol. 12, No. 2, pp. 238–49.

Payne, S. (1997) 'Nursing research: a social science?', in McKenzie, G., Powell, J. and Usher, R. (eds) *Understanding Social Research: Perspectives on Methodology and Practice*, pp. 101–11, London, Falmer Press.

Ribeaux, P. and Spence, M. (2001) 'CAM evaluation: what are the research questions?', *Complementary Therapies in Medicine*, Vol. 9, pp. 188–93.

Ribeiro, V. (2002) 'Review: some herbal medicines and plant extracts reduced pain and disability and improved function in osteoarthritis', *Evidence-Based Nursing*, Vol. 5, No. 2, p. 57.

Risberg T., Vickers, A., Bremnes, R., Wist, E., Kaasa, S. and Cassileth, B. (2002) 'Does use of alternative medicine predict survival from cancer?', *European Journal of Cancer*, Vol. 39, No. 3, pp. 372–7.

Shah, A. and Dickenson, D. (1999) 'The capacity to make decisions in dementia: some contemporary issues', *International Journal of Geriatric Psychiatry*, Vol. 14, pp. 803–6.

Stux, G. and Hammerschlag, R. (eds) (2000) *Clinical Acupuncture: Scientific Basis*, Berlin, Springer.

Taggart, H. M., Arslanian, C. L., Bae, S. and Singh, K. (2003) 'Effects of T'ai Chi exercise on fibromyalgia symptoms and health-related quality of life', *Orthopaedic Nursing*, Vol. 22, No. 5, pp. 353–60.

Thomas, K. and Fitter, M. (2002) 'Possible research strategies for evaluating CAM interventions', in Lewith, G., Jonas, W. B. and Walach, H. (eds) *Clinical Research in Complementary Therapies*, London, Churchill Livingstone.

Verhoef, M. J., Casebeer, A. L. and Hilsden, M. D. (2002) 'Assessing efficacy of complementary medicine: adding qualitative research methods to the "Gold Standard"', *The Journal of Alternative and Complementary Medicine*, Vol. 8, No. 3, pp. 275–81.

Vickers, A. J., Rees, R. W., Zollman, C. E., McCarney, R., Smith, C., Ellis, N., Fisher, P. and Van Haselen, R. (2004) 'Acupuncture for chronic headache in primary care: large, pragmatic, randomised trial', *British Medical Journal*, Vol. 328, pp. 744–9.

Ware, J. E. and Sherbourne, C. D. (1992) 'The MOS 36-item Short-Form Health Survey (SF-36). Conceptual framework and item selection', *Medical Care*, Vol. 30, pp. 473–83.

Wassern, R., McDonald, M. and Racine, J. (2002) 'Fibromyalgia: patient perspectives on symptoms, symptom management, and provider utilization', *Clinical Nurse Specialist*, Vol. 76, No. 1, pp. 24–28.

Wenneberg, S., Gunnarsson, L. G. and Ahlström, G. (2004) 'Using a novel exercise programme for patients with muscular dystrophy. Part I: a qualitative study', *Disability and Rehabilitation*, Vol. 26, No. 10, pp. 586–94.

Wigers, S., Stiles, T. and Vogel, P. (1966) 'Effects of aerobic exercise versus stress management treatment in fibromyalgia', *Scandinavian Journal of Rheumatology*, Vol. 25, pp. 77–86.

Wiles, A. and Booker, D. (2005) 'Complementary therapies in dementia care', in Lee-Treweek, G., Heller, T. and Spurr, S. (eds) *Perspectives on Complementary and Alternative Medicine: A Reader*, pp. 379–90, Abingdon, Routledge/The Open University (K221 Set Book).

Wolfe, F., Ross, K., Anderson, J., Russell, I. J. and Hobert, L. (1995) 'The prevalence and characteristics of fibromyalgia in the general population', *Arthritis and Rheumatism*, Vol. 38, pp. 19–28.

Chapter 9 Evaluating practice in complementary and alternative medicine

Tom Heller, Dione Hills and Elaine Weatherley-Jones

Contents

AIMS

- To give an overview of the ways in which health projects and services can be evaluated.
- To explore the issues in evaluating CAM provision.
- To describe practical examples of evaluation methods that are relevant to CAM projects.

9.1 Introduction

This chapter discusses how practice in complementary and alternative medicine (CAM) can be evaluated. This is distinctly different from attempts to prove or disprove whether particular CAM interventions are effective for specific conditions, which was the subject of Chapter 8. Evaluation cannot determine the efficacy of individual treatments or therapies, but it can shed light on the practice of CAM within a specific setting or project. The following quotation applies to both research and evaluation:

> The history of evaluation research teaches us that there is no such thing as the right method, the best method or the gold standard of research. There is only good research applied to a relevant question with the appropriate

consideration of measurement and socially skillful manipulation of the results. It is only the multiplicity of methods and the variety of approaches, as well as complementary skills of the researcher, which will help us solve the questions in front of us.

(Wittmann and Walach, 2002, p. 106)

There is no single, agreed, simple definition of what an evaluation is. It can also be difficult to clarify the distinctions between evaluation, research and audit. **Research** in the context of health and social care usually aims to establish what is **best practice**. It is often designed to be replicated and so that its results can be generalised to other similar situations. It aims to generate new knowledge or increase the sum of knowledge. Research is usually initiated by the researchers and may be theory driven. In a clinical or therapeutic setting, **audit** usually involves systematically looking at the procedures used for diagnosis, care and treatment; examining how the associated resources are used; and investigating the effect care has on the outcome and quality of life for people having that treatment or taking part in the project being audited. **Evaluation**, which is the main focus of this chapter, includes the systematic empirical examination of a service or a social programme's design, implementation and impacts with a view to judging its merit, worth and significance. Evaluation usually reduces uncertainty for people making decisions about the service, helps facilitate service improvement and often serves a political function.

There is no need to restrict the type of inquiry that is undertaken: several different types of study may be used within one service. For example, if the intention is to find out more about an in-patient unit for people with eating disorders, a study that considers whether the people admitted to the unit benefited most from group or individual psychotherapy would be **research**. However, a study that examines whether the following standard set by the staff on the unit was being achieved – 'All people admitted to the unit will receive a team assessment within two days of admission to decide whether they should receive group or individual psychotherapy' – is a **clinical audit** project. Grabowska et al. (2003) describe an example of a clinical audit. In addition, a study involving (a) collecting information about service users to see whether the service is reaching the target population and (b) obtaining feedback from service users and referrers about various aspects of the service (for example, accessibility) is a service **evaluation**. Several examples of evaluation are considered in this chapter.

Focus on evaluation

Evaluation usually involves applying methods and knowledge of social science in order to make rational and well informed decisions about programmes of intervention (Shadish et al., 1991). This is as true for

CAM-related evaluation as for different types of evaluation in a more general context. The concept of evaluation became popular during the 1960s in the USA, when social programmes were developed to promote social welfare through educational investment and other forms of social intervention. Obviously, those making the investment wanted a way of finding out whether what they were doing, or at least paying for, was having any effect.

Scriven (1991, p. 139) suggests that the term 'evaluation' is most widely used to refer to the process of determining the merit, worth or value of something, or the product of that process. In his opinion, the evaluation process normally involves: some identification of relevant standards of merit, worth or value; some investigation of the performance of people being evaluated against these standards; and some integration or synthesis of the results to achieve an overall evaluation.

Although there is a growing tendency to use the term 'evaluation' to describe only the most formal types of study, this could overlook the amount of ongoing, self-evaluative activities that are built into many projects and programmes. Having specific points for reflection and self-evaluation is generally regarded as good practice, particularly in new and experimental projects and programmes. Many CAM practitioners have a period of time for evaluation and reflection built in to their working practices. Although these kinds of self-evaluation activity may be criticised as 'unscientific', they can include considerable amounts of systematic data collection and analysis and they certainly are important to the people doing the work.

This criticism of some informal types of evaluation may arise from confusion between the concepts of evaluation and research, and from assumptions about what kind of research questions and research methods are valid and acceptable. Although there is no hard-and-fast line between research and evaluation, the central concern in research is to produce knowledge that is generalisable (Scriven, 1991); while evaluation, within CAM and elsewhere, is more concerned with deriving learning from a particular setting or programme. There is also the matter of **judgement**: while evaluation involves judgement against previously determined criteria, in research, data are usually compared with a set of hypotheses, which have generally been derived from theory, and strenuous attempts are made to ensure objectivity and neutrality that may not be appropriate in a CAM environment.

9.2   Why carry out an evaluation?

There are many different reasons for evaluating a CAM-related treatment or service. These reasons will help determine the kind of evaluation questions asked, as well as the methodology chosen. Chelimsky (1997) clusters the reasons for doing evaluations under the headings 'accountability', 'development' and 'knowledge'. Using this scheme, **accountability** is the reason for evaluation when it is primarily used to provide evidence that funding or grants have been used to good effect: for example, when integrating CAM therapies with NHS services. **Development** infers that evaluation could be used to help strengthen institutions or CAM programmes, learning from detailed study of the parts of the work that went well or those where changes are needed. The **knowledge** base of evaluation is helpful in obtaining a deeper understanding of a specific area or policy that relates to CAM.

Evaluations in the CAM tradition may be done for some or all of these reasons, although most will focus primarily on one. However, there may be confusion about what the primary purpose is, particularly if the people involved are not explicit about their intentions, or there is disagreement among them. For example, a new service might be evaluated as a condition of funding, for the purposes of accountability; at the same time, it might be 'sold' to the service provider as being useful for the development of the service. However, if the results are subsequently written up for publication and submitted to a medical research journal rather than one with a more general audience, or a CAM-specific journal, it might be criticised for failing to use methodology that could provide generalisable findings.

The need for evaluation strategies that were linked closely with a specific purpose was one of the main driving forces behind Quinn Patton's 'utilisation-focused evaluation' (1986). Although this was developed for a general audience, the relevance for CAM is apparent. He suggested, among other things, that:

- Evaluations should be user-orientated, i.e. aimed at the interest and information needs of specific, identifiable people, not vague, passive audiences.
- Various factors can affect use: community variables, organisational characteristics, the nature of the evaluator, evaluator credibility, political considerations and resource constraints. The evaluator needs to be sensitive to and aware of how various factors and conditions affect the potential use of the evaluation.
- There are multiple and varied interests: the process of identifying and organising stakeholders to participate in an evaluation process should be done in a way that is sensitive to and respectful of these varied and multiple interests.
- Evaluators committed to enhancing utilisation have a responsibility to train stakeholders in the evaluation process and the uses of information.

Wittmann and Walach (2002) make a similar plea specifically in the context of CAM-related research and evaluation as follows.

Results of research studies in CAM are never just bland facts. They are always facts for an audience, facts in favor of or against practical decisions. It is wise to have possible audiences in view right from the start of a study. Thus, if a study is meant to address purchasers or political decision makers, it is wise to consider what type of information is going to impress them ... for political authorities or health-care decision makers sound scientific evidence of statistical superiority of a treatment over control might be mandatory, for purchasers it could be enough to demonstrate a certain level of practical usefulness.

(Wittmann and Walach, 2002, pp. 105–6)

9.3   The stakeholders in an evaluation

The term 'stakeholders' generally means groups within a programme or project who have a different 'stake' or interest in its activities. For example, Barr et al. (2000) identify three groups of stakeholders in most evaluations of community health projects: programme sponsors, programme workers and programme consumers. Note the absence from this list of the wider audience of policy makers or academics, who require 'evidence' of effectiveness for future policy developments, and researchers, who might want an evaluation out of professional interest or to advance their academic career.

As Table 9.1 shows, the interests of stakeholders do not always coincide, and there may be considerable tension within a programme between the different evaluation requirements of each group. These various purposes can manifest themselves in a commitment to different evaluation questions and different strategies. This is why anyone doing an evaluation in a CAM setting must discuss their plans with representatives from different stakeholder groups, before finalising their design.

TABLE 9.1 STAKEHOLDERS AND THEIR INTERESTS IN EVALUATION	
Parties with an interest in evaluation	**Motives for evaluation**
Programme sponsors: local authorities, central government, trusts, professional bodies for therapists, etc.	Political accountability for funding Decisions for future funding Lessons for future policy and programmes
Programme workers: field staff and managers	Improving competitiveness in funding market Lessons for future development of practice Personal learning about skills and techniques
Programme consumers: patients, community members, other agencies, etc.	Lessons for future action Interest in the success of the project Personal learning for the future

ACTIVITY   EVALUATING CAM APPROACHES IN PRIMARY CARE

Allow 45 minutes

Read the extract in Box 9.1 from the report of an evaluation of a primary care project that explored some people's experience of using CAM and its impact on their physical and mental health and wellbeing. This study by Stella Carmichael (2003) aimed to give an insight into the perceived impact of CAM on the health and wellbeing of a small but representative group of people living in a disadvantaged area of Newcastle upon Tyne. As you read the report, consider the following questions.

1   In your opinion, why was this particular evaluation carried out?

2   Who would you consider to be the key 'stakeholders' in this project?

3   What potential impact do you think this evaluation might have on the stakeholders?

BOX 9.1   CAM AND PRIMARY CARE: AN EVALUATION

A three-year project was funded by Newcastle Primary Care Team to pilot a model of integration of complementary therapies alongside orthodox medical approaches. To enable integration between complementary medicine and primary care, a number of complementary practitioners were based at general practitioner (GP) surgeries. Patients could be referred by their own GP to any of the surgeries hosting complementary practitioners. The following treatments were available: acupuncture, aromatherapy, chiropractic, homeopathy, osteopathy and shiatsu. Patients living in the area could also make a self-referral.

It was agreed that qualitative research would provide a greater understanding of why people chose to try CAM, and its perceived impact. Interviews were used to explore patients' experiences. Particular emphasis was given to the perceived effects on their mental health and wellbeing.

A purposive sample of patients were targeted for interview, ensuring there was equal representation for all the therapies offered in the service.

Methodology

This research was carried out from a feminist perspective which encourages a person-centred approach, enabling the individual's values and opinions to be voiced, and validates their perception of their own health. It also acknowledges the importance of the relationship between the interviewer and the interviewee.

The interviews consisted of semi-structured, open-ended questions and lasted up to an hour. They were recorded and then transcribed by a professional transcription service. A rigorous approach was taken when analysing the transcriptions using 'grounded theory' (Strauss and Corbin, 1990), which allows inherent themes to emerge from the collected interview data. Grounded theory is a methodology used by researchers and evaluators to develop their understanding of a situation through a series of stages and checks. After any information is gathered it is checked against information from other sources until a theory or an understanding emerges that fits with all the collected data.

Results

The interviews found the majority of people felt there had been an improvement in their physical health, and over half of all participants felt there had been an improvement in their mental health.

■ All of these patients shared a common goal: to achieve an improvement in their own health and wellbeing. People clearly want to be involved in their own health care, and when they were this proved to be an empowering experience.

■ Whether people were trying complementary medicine for the first time or whether they had previous experience, a key factor in its success was attributed to the therapist's approach and ability to listen.

■ The improvements people hoped to gain from the treatments were realistic: only one person expected to find a cure for their chronic condition. Where there was early intervention the improvement was much greater and sometimes permanent.

■ For many, the relief from pain enabled greater participation in daily activities, and this seemed to correlate with a more positive mental state. The inability to partake in normal activities can lead to social exclusion. Social exclusion has been identified as a cause of mental health problems as well as a symptom. Even though this is an evaluation of the service and not a research project to determine the efficacy of CAM interventions it is of great interest that CAM was effective in reducing the pain experienced by participants of the service.

■ Integration with the NHS was seen as a very positive association, it gave many patients the confidence to try complementary medicine in the first place. The GP surgery was the favoured place to access complementary medicine as long as it wasn't too far away, or too difficult to travel to.

■ Complementary medicine was considered an alternative to medication. Given the choice the majority of patients said they would prefer not to take any medication at all because of unwanted side effects.

■ Offering a choice of complementary and alternative therapy treatments and having the flexibility to refer a patient to more than one therapy enabled people to find a treatment that worked best for them.

■ Patients clearly found CAM to be of real and long-term benefit in the relief of pain and stress, leading to an improvement for most in their mental health and wellbeing. From the patients' perspective most have felt improvements in their health that far outweigh any improvements that orthodox medicine alone has been able to achieve for the long-term suffering of the medical conditions they were referred with. All but one person would try CAM again and hoped that it would continue to be available.

(Source: adapted from Carmichael, 2003)

Comment

1 Evaluation might have been a specific requirement of the organisation that funds the service: 'If you can't show that it's effective, we won't give you any further funding.' For other projects the motive may be less pragmatic and more focused on the need to use the evaluation results to make further improvements in the project itself.

2 Although the term 'stakeholders' may be considered modern jargon that is used (and misused) in many recent official documents, considering all the people affected by a particular project, 'stakeholders' could be a very useful term. The case in the report in Box 9.1 might be considered to have many potential 'stakeholders', including grant-giving agencies; local development agencies; Primary Care Team officers and board members; local GPs and other primary care workers; and members of the local community, including those who represent all the relevant ethnic minority groups. You probably thought of many other people who could have been consulted in the design and implementation of any evaluation of the project and with whom the results of the evaluation should be shared: for example, the 'expert patient' groups or those associated with support for people with particular health problems.

3 If the evaluation does highlight problems within the service, or signal ways of improving it, this is a powerful motivator for continuing with regular evaluations.

9.4 What is being evaluated?

Evaluation can be used to assess the impact of not only specific CAM treatments but also more particularly how treatments are being delivered to people who attend for treatment, or their contribution to 'quality of life' (for example, in palliative care), or very importantly, client satisfaction. One of the most frequent demands for evaluation arises when people want to establish a new 'integrated' service, in which CAM therapies are used to complement orthodox treatments. It is important, therefore, to be clear about what is the key aspect that is being evaluated: a specific treatment, or a combination of treatments, or the service as a whole.

The evaluation questions in each case might be very different. In an individual CAM treatment, the questions might focus on alleviating certain unpleasant symptoms. For a set of treatments, the question might be about their overall contribution to people's quality of life. Evaluation may also concern broader questions about the integration of the therapies: the effectiveness and appropriateness of referrals, or the level of communication between health professionals. Another example is the use of complementary therapies as part of a wider programme of health promotion: for example, in a 'healthy living' centre. In this case, the complementary therapy might be used to attract people to attend the centre, from which they could be channelled into other activities.

Thomas and Fitter (2002) list the following three main approaches for evaluating CAM interventions and in Box 9.2 their links with specific research questions.

1 **Proving studies**: designed to provide definitive information about efficacy, effectiveness and safety. Proving studies are divided into efficacy (randomised controlled trials), comparative effectiveness (e.g. pragmatic RCTs, patient preference studies, economic evaluation, cost-effectiveness studies) and evidence review (systematic review, meta-analysis).

2 **Exploratory studies**: often smaller and less definitive, they contribute to the pool of information and provide the groundwork for making decisions about a full study. Examples are pilot studies and clinical outcome studies.

3 **Improving studies**: are rooted in everyday practice, and aim to improve practice through greater understanding of the clinical process and its components. Examples include reflective and clinical practice, such as case studies and diagnostic concordance studies, and service delivery evaluations, including co-operative inquiry and action research studies.

BOX 9.2   WAYS OF EVALUATING CAM PRACTICE AND THEIR RELEVANT RESEARCH QUESTIONS

Proving studies

Efficacy

- Is there a specific beneficial effect?
- What is the active ingredient?

Comparative effectiveness

- How well does it work in practice?
- How does it compare with other treatments or services?

Economic evaluation

- Is it value for money?

Evidence review

- What do we already know?
- What does the cumulative evidence tell us?
- What further studies are needed?

Exploratory studies

- Does this procedure appear to be safe and offer benefits?
- Is there sufficient evidence of benefit to justify a full trial?
- What are the appropriate outcome measures?
- Is a trial feasible?

(continued)

> ### *Improving studies*
>
> *Reflective and clinical practice*
>
> - Can I improve my practice through monitoring and reflecting on practice?
> - Is this diagnostic procedure valid and reliable?
> - Can use of a diagnostic test result in more cost-effectively targeted services?
>
> *Service delivery*
>
> - Is this new service effective in the wider service framework within which it has been established?
> - What factors are enabling or impeding effective organisation and delivery of services?
>
> (Source: adapted from Thomas and Fitter, 2002, pp. 62–3, 75, 80–1)

9.5   Planning an evaluation

Deciding on research variables

A key prerequisite when planning an evaluation is to decide which variables to include. The appropriate variables depend on two questions: first, why is the evaluation needed and, second, who is it for? These are questions about the purpose or reason for the evaluation as well as the stakeholders or interested parties. Three overarching reasons were identified in Section 9.2: accountability, development and contribution to the knowledge base. Closely related to the reasons for doing an evaluation is the question of stakeholders or those for whom the evaluation is being done. In Table 9.1 three groups were suggested: programme sponsors, programme workers and programme consumers. In many ways these groups fit with the reasons identified: programme sponsors are likely to be concerned with accountability; programme workers with developing the service; and programme consumers with gaining a better insight into the knowledge base.

An evaluation that could satisfy all the stakeholders and fulfil the three main reasons for doing it needs to pay attention not just to the outcomes of the service or therapy to be evaluated but also to the processes involved in providing that service or therapy. Ribeaux and Spence (2001) see this as key to evaluating CAM in a holistic way that does justice to the full complexity of the CAM experience. They argue that evaluating the therapist as well as the therapy and the user is vital to understanding the process of delivering CAM therapies: 'evaluation of the therapist may provide a relevant solution to the evaluation of CAM therapies since often the treatment variables are assembled on a patient by patient basis by the therapist' (p. 192).

TABLE 9.2 RESEARCH VARIABLES IN EVALUATING DELIVERY AND OUTCOME OF CAM THERAPIES	
Therapist	**Patient**
Process variables	
Background: training (who with, for how long), experience with the therapy, additional CAM training (in other therapies), reasons for practising the specific therapy	Background: demographic data (age, education, income), experience with CAM in general, experience with specific therapy, health history
Philosophy: practitioners' beliefs concerning the scope of the therapy	Philosophy: life style, personal philosophy, ways of approaching life in general
Expectations: vis-à-vis individual patients	Expectations: vis-à-vis the specific therapy
Techniques: reasons for using the various techniques, methods, approaches, words, touch, look, tone of voice, etc.	Reasons for using the specific therapy, involvement with the process
Experience with the patient and the way the techniques were received	Experience with the therapist and the therapy
Outcome variables	
Objective measures of therapist credentials: qualifications, years of experience, types of conditions treated, self-development through attendance at conferences, etc.	Objective measures of medical condition: blood pressure, joint mobility, etc.
Satisfaction with the interaction with the patient, with the progress the patient has made	Satisfaction with the therapist, the therapy, the advice given, the progress experienced; change in symptoms

(Source: Ribeaux and Spence, 2001, p. 191, Table 2)

Ribeaux and Spence (2001) suggest several process and outcome variables from the perspective of both therapist and user ('patient') which should be involved in evaluating a CAM therapy (see Table 9.2).

Different methods are appropriate for evaluating these different aspects of process and outcome. Ribeaux and Spence believe that 'this is a place where art meets science and requires creative use of research techniques' (2001, p. 192). They suggest that qualitative techniques are more suited to developing holistic measures of therapy delivery as well as subjective measures of outcomes such as patient satisfaction. More scientific objective measures would be appropriate for assessing outcomes such as improvement in medical condition.

Chapter 7 discussed how one of the difficulties in CAM research and evaluation has been the use of inquiry methods that practitioners believe are not sympathetic to the nature of how they work. Examples include selecting only one aspect of the treatment, whereas in fact the usual CAM treatment may involve a range of interventions; or selecting one method – such as using a specific acupuncture point – where, in reality, this point is only used with some of the people who have a particular problem and where, in practice, most acupuncture is based on tailoring specific treatments to the particular person who attends for treatment. Combining methods and evaluating CAM therapies in the holistic way suggested by Ribeaux and Spence should help address some of the concerns of CAM practitioners.

Unfortunately, many evaluations are driven by stakeholders, such as funders, who are only interested in outcome measures. The holistic evaluation of process and outcome suggested by Ribeaux and Spence can be expensive and time-consuming. So it is important to take account of the resources that are available for any evaluation.

Availability of resources

The resources available for evaluating a CAM project or programme are often limited, which can be an important factor in deciding on the type of evaluation. In CAM, resources and energy for evaluation may be considered a low priority when competing for scarce resources. Trying to undertake a study that either requires a considerable input of time or money (for example, in postage for questionnaires and responses) or has problems in getting people with the necessary skills for analysing data can lead to frustration and, often, unfavourable evaluation results. If the evaluation was conducted under less than ideal conditions, they should be clearly outlined in the evaluation report itself.

Unless the evaluation is self-evaluation, the necessary resources for collecting data and disseminating results should be in place. Sufficient time and funding are required to ensure that the evaluation produces valid results:

> cost-cutting is likely to produce studies that have a serious risk of either answering an inappropriate question, or having little chance *a priori* of providing an adequate answer to a relevant question.
>
> (White and Hart, 2002, p. 60)

Time

It is necessary to consider the time required both for the evaluation activities and for gathering enough data. The amount of time allocated must be sufficient for the requisite numbers of people with a particular condition to have access to the service. The time it will probably take before there is a change in a condition or service provision should never be underestimated. For example, in some cases, it is useful to follow up people receiving treatment for 12 months or more.

Money

Apart from the fact that, as far as therapists are concerned, time is money, some aspects of research or evaluation can be quite expensive. For example, access to literature, validated tests and software for analysing data can be expensive, as are the printing and postage costs of sending out large numbers of questionnaires and reminders.

Skill

This is often an underestimated resource. Those doing the evaluation need to have either experience themselves of or access to advice on evaluation design, use of suitable methods, data analysis and report writing.

Background knowledge and experience

It is advisable for the person or team doing the evaluation to have some experience of the therapy being evaluated, or to have direct access to people with this experience who can give ongoing advice about the research method. It is also very important to have reviewed other published research in the field before starting: there is no point in duplicating what someone else has done if the aim is to contribute to the knowledge base. If a specific service is being evaluated, it is always useful to know what other researchers have done beforehand.

Client input

Involving the people under treatment in research design is increasingly seen to be good practice in health service and clinical research (Boote et al., 2002; Telford et al., 2002). For example, in the UK the organisation called INVOLVE promotes public involvement in NHS, public health and social care research (INVOLVE, 2004).

Being appropriate to the treatment, project or programme

The evaluation method chosen needs to be appropriate, not only to the questions being asked but also to the health intervention, or service, itself.

ACTIVITY   EVALUATING A MENOPAUSE CLINIC THAT USES CAM

Allow 45 minutes

Read the extract in Box 9.3 from a report by Thomas et al. (2001) of an evaluation of a menopause clinic that uses CAM.

After you have read the report, answer the following questions.

1   Who were the 'stakeholders' in this evaluation and which particular results might they be interested in?

2   What were the outcomes in terms of the effectiveness of treatment in helping women with menopausal symptoms?

3   What were the process outcomes in terms of running the service?

BOX 9.3   CAM AND A MENOPAUSE CLINIC: AN EVALUATION

An NHS Menopause Clinic offers two types of CAM (homeopathy and aromatherapy). This newly expanded complementary therapy service is funded by a service development award from the Community Trust.

Aims of the evaluation

To assess how far the CAM service is able to operate successfully within the menopause clinic, and offer beneficial treatment to patients who might not otherwise receive homeopathy or aromatherapy. Beneficial treatment was defined as a measurable reduction of self-reported symptoms associated with the menopause.

There is considerable demand for CAM interventions and little evidence on which to base such decisions. The results from the service evaluation were intended to help inform future NHS commissioning decisions.

A service evaluation was undertaken using a combination of qualitative and quantitative methods. A validated outcome measure — Measure Yourself Medical Outcome Profile (MYMOP; Paterson, 1996) — was employed to assess patient responses to treatment and treatment outcomes. Service provider and patient perspectives were elicited using semi-structured interviews, and a postal survey.

MYMOP data were collected and recorded at baseline for 58 patients out of the 77 for which records were available (75%). The 54 patients for whom there were outcome data were similar to the whole population of patients with respect to age (mean 50.5 years), menopausal status and HRT use. The average MYMOP scores reduced significantly between the baseline and the sixth or final visit for women whether they were treated by homeopaths or by aromatherapists.

These positive results indicate that the CAM service at the Clinic was associated with clearly identifiable short-term positive benefits in the control of menopausal symptoms as detected by the MYMOP measure.

Practitioner perspectives were sought about how the process of working together had evolved and the lessons learnt that could be of help to other such services. Four of the key practitioners involved were interviewed (3 complementary, 1 orthodox). The interviews were all conducted using a semi-structured interview schedule. All the practitioners were very pleased with the service and felt that it had brought benefits to both patients and themselves. The practitioners felt that the complementary therapy service had worked well alongside conventional treatment, as one said: 'it's very much integrated medicine', in the sense that both the homeopathy and aromatherapy were working alongside the conventional treatments, like HRT, that the clinic provided.

Analysis of the interviews also identified that, in establishing the service, it took a considerable period for the referral system to be sorted out. Initially the complementary practitioners were seeing a wide range of patients, many not with menopausal symptoms. One practitioner felt that the service was initially 'used slightly as a dumping ground' for patients who had proved difficult to treat conventionally. The orthodox practitioner admitted that it had been 'chaos' at the beginning, when clients could self-refer. The range of patients being seen and demand for the service led to the development of a clear protocol for referral which was felt to have resulted both in a steady flow of appropriate patients and a way of curtailing high demand for the service.

(Source: adapted from Thomas et al., 2001)

Comment

1   The main stakeholders in the evaluation of this project seem to be the funding organisation, the people running the service, the workers within the service and, of course, the women attending the clinic.

2   The Community Trust, which makes a grant towards providing the service, will be interested to discover whether the service they are paying for responds to people's perceived health care needs. The service providers — the organisers of the menopause clinic — will want to use the evaluation to discover whether the CAM service can operate successfully within the menopause clinic. The practitioners will be interested in the process of integrated working as well as the outcomes of their treatment. The people attending the service will be especially concerned about the outcomes of treatment.

3   The process of doing the evaluation appears to have led to the development of a protocol for using the service which, in turn, provided 'a way of curtailing high demand for the service'. Of course, this could be questioned as a positive outcome of the evaluation. On the one hand, it has exposed considerable satisfaction with the service but, on the other, it has resulted in a way of reducing or controlling demand for this service from people with significant symptoms.

9.6   Quality criteria in an evaluation

Traditionally, the quality of mainstream evaluations is judged primarily in terms of the adequacy of the investigation design and its methodology in terms of whether it answered the question addressed. However, in the world of CAM-related evaluation, the quality of the methodology used is only one of several criteria that need to be considered. In various standards for evaluation that have been established by associations of evaluators, different dimensions have been identified which apply to both CAM and orthodox situations. For example, Box 9.4 (overleaf) shows the American Evaluation Association's guiding principles for evaluators.

BOX 9.4 GUIDING PRINCIPLES FOR EVALUATORS

1 **Systematic inquiry**: evaluators conduct systematic, data-based inquiries about whatever is being evaluated.

2 **Competence**: evaluators provide competent performance to stakeholders.

3 **Integrity/honesty**: evaluators ensure the honesty and integrity of the entire evaluation process.

4 **Respect for people**: evaluators respect the security, dignity and self-worth of the respondents, program participants, clients, and other stakeholders with whom they interact.

5 **Responsibilities for general and public welfare**: evaluators articulate and take into account the diversity of interests and values that may be related to the general and public welfare.

(Source: American Evaluation Association, 1994)

ACTIVITY EVALUATING A COMMUNITY HEALTH PROJECT THAT USES CAM

Allow 1 hour

Read the report in Box 9.5 of an evaluation of a community-based project, which aimed to provide a picture of demand for CAM in a specific area of East Bristol (Monk and Chaplin, 2002). After reading the report, try to answer the following questions.

1 Imagine that you are a philanthropic lottery winner who is considering investing some of your winnings in a project such as this one. Using the criteria listed in Box 9.6 (page 251), what would you want to know about the project before handing over a large cheque that enabled it to continue?

2 Do you think that the evaluation helps you to reach a decision about how you should spend your money?

3 What additional questions would you like answered when evaluating such a project?

BOX 9.5 AN EVALUATION OF THE COMMUNITY HEALTH IN PARTNERSHIPS PROJECT

This report is from an overview and evaluation of the Community Health in Partnerships (CHIPS) Pilot Project from June 2001 to March 2002. It aims to provide a picture of the demand for the CHIPS project and the impact it has made in the New Deal for Communities (NDC) area in East Bristol.

The NDC is a key programme in the Government's strategy to help some of the most deprived neighbourhoods in the country. Programmes are formulated and delivered through partnerships formed between local people, community and voluntary organisations, public agencies, local authorities and local businesses.

As part of the sustainable health and wellbeing outcome area, which is one part of the NDC agenda, a group of local community workers and complementary therapists formed a Steering Group in the summer of 2000 and started to work up a funding bid and work plan to develop a project which would provide complementary health services locally – focusing on employing local unemployed therapists and charging low treatment costs which would be largely subsidised.

Following the success of the first pilot, the CHIPS project applied for and was awarded an extension to continue the service, providing: a safe, qualified and quality service for local people; opportunities for funding partnerships to undertake primary care research; and opportunities to work in partnership with practices in the area to develop an integrated health service into the longer term.

Project Aims

- To continue to deliver CHIPS services to local residents at a new 40–50 treatments a week target
- To monitor the full impact of the initial pilot (July 2001 to March 2002)
- To introduce nutrition to the range of support offered
- To employ a local resident as a part-time CHIPS Support Worker to assist with bookings and project systems
- To identify a local CHIPS base: office, equipment storage and therapy location
- To develop a two-year 'bridging' project for CHIPS 2002–2004 until the launch of the Healthy Living Centre and identify funding partnerships (social and medical)

Project Activities

- Undertake 40 treatments each week for the first 4 months, and 50 treatments each week in the last 4 months of the project: reflexology; aromatherapy; massage; shiatsu; acupuncture; acupressure; osteopathy; and nutrition
- Continue to deliver treatments from Lawrence Hill Health Centre, Corbett House Surgery, Corbett House Clinic and Community Around Alcohol and Drugs project
- Client certification to provide cheaper treatments to those local residents in receipt of benefit (£5 waged; £3 concessionary)
- Recruit a local resident at 16 hrs Administrative Grade (£12,618–£13,500) as a CHIPS Project Support Worker
- Recruit new lead and reserve nutritionists
- Develop a more effective booking system for the project in liaison with therapists/surgeries

- Develop joint work with 9 projects across Community at Heart
- Establish a GP/Health Professional consultative group to develop project protocol and strengthen medical relations
- Identify and establish a CHIPS base for an office, resource library, equipment store, and therapy room. This will free-up CAH [Community at Heart] management and administration office space, and will allow CHIPS to develop its own therapy space for community use
- Contact similar complementary health schemes in NDC across the UK and Health Action Zones to do best practice research and inform future fundraising and development proposals
- Manage the Community at Heart staff Stress Management Service
- Network and fundraise to develop a two-year 'bridging' project in partnership with Healthy Bristol around more clinical based research
- To identify target patient groups to research the impact of complementary health on medical intervention and well-being (e.g. back pain, stress and anxiety conditions)
- Strengthen monitoring systems and establish a Users Group to help feed into the process

Did we achieve our aims?

- **To continue to deliver CHIPS services to local residents at a new 40–50 treatments a week target** With the new dedicated CHIPS therapy room in the Portakabin at the back of Corbett Surgery, CHIPS has been able to deliver up to 50 treatments per week.
- **To monitor the full impact of the initial pilot (July 2001 to March 2002)** The report evaluated in depth the impact of the initial pilot using data from the First and Last Treatment Forms that CHIPS clients are asked to complete.
- **To introduce nutrition to the range of support offered** Nutrition was successfully introduced in May 2002.
- **To employ a local resident as a part-time CHIPS Support Worker to assist with bookings and project systems** There were no applications for the part-time CHIPS Support Worker post. Therefore the post was revised and became a full-time HPHP Project Support Worker post, half of whose time to be spent on CHIPS work. A local resident started work with the project on 10 June 2002.
- **To identify a local CHIPS base: office, equipment storage and therapy location** CHIPS is now located in the Portakabin off Corbett House Surgery. CHIPS shares an office with the CAH Health Development Manager and has a dedicated therapy room in the Portakabin from which to deliver its services.
- **To develop a two-year 'bridging' project for CHIPS 2002–2004 until the launch of the Healthy Living Centre and identify funding partnerships (social and medical)** CHIPS has successfully bid for a

three-year (rather than two-year) bridging project, mainly funded by CAH. It is hoped that this 'bridging' project will give CHIPS enough time to secure long-term funding.

Impact of Therapies on Health of Clients

Following the first pilot, CHIPS was able to measure the impact of its work on clients through asking clients to mark themselves on a scale of 1 to 10 (where 1 is bad) according to how they felt in terms of their:

- immunity
- energy levels
- stress levels
- sleep patterns
- physical health
- emotional health
- mental health
- pain levels.

This question was asked at both their first and last treatments in order to see where improvements had been made. The following results have been calculated from the client questionnaires [a total of 1620 treatments over the course of the eight-month project]:

- 93% reported a reduction in stress levels
- 89% reported an improvement in their sleep patterns
- 89% reported a reduction in physical pain
- 86% of clients reported an improvement in the strength of their immunity
- 86% reported an improvement in their overall physical health
- 82% reported an improvement in emotional health
- 82% reported an improvement in mental health
- 79% of clients reported an improvement in energy levels.

Following treatment, 14% of clients reported that their symptoms had ceased or became significantly milder than before treatment.

Case Reports

A number of CHIPS clients reported that the treatment they received was so beneficial they wanted to write 'their story' for this study. In addition to this, all therapists were asked to compile a 'typical' case study from their pilot clients.

What has the pilot shown us?

- **The need for comprehensive policies and procedures** In particular around bookings, such as how many each client can receive, how a client is allocated to a therapy, should we have priority ratings, etc.
- **The need to educate local GPs and health workers around each therapy** Following discussions at the GP liaison meetings and CHIPS

Research Group meetings, the GPs have expressed their limited knowledge of what each therapy involves and can offer; this is reflected in the fact that 52% of their referrals to the project were for Osteopathy alone. It is envisaged that training sessions will be organised for local health professionals run by Healthy Bristol in partnership with CHIPS. Such sessions would include: the holistic vision and an insight into each therapy; the procedures involved, their benefits, the training that therapists undertake, etc. From these, it is hoped that they will have a greater understanding of the therapies offered and what conditions they are helpful in, as well as a greater confidence in referring people with a wider variety of symptoms to the project.

- **The need for additional staffing hours** The workload of the project has increased much in recent months as monitoring demands from CAH grow and involvement in development work has increased. CHIPS currently has one 0.5 project support worker post and one 0.8 project co-ordinator post.

- **The need for a more workable and efficient booking and monitoring system** It has been increasingly frustrating the amount of people hours that goes into bookings and gathering data from the project such as DNA's, number of bookings. Various avenues have been looked at but none to date have suited the needs of the project, which would be within our budget. It is thought that an ideal system would be computerised and that the various data that we collect can more easily be inputted, and monitoring data extracted, without the need for paper counting! Such a system is vital if we are to more comprehensively monitor the project in the future, as planned.

- **The importance of keeping abreast of national best practice and policy** Our involvement with the Prince of Wales's Foundation for Integrated Health and the many links this has facilitated, has shown how useful it is for a project such as CHIPS, at the forefront of changing health service policy, to link with others and find out policy changes and best practice, both to continually improve our service to local residents as well as assisting with the all important task of making the project much more appealing to future funders.

- **The need to break down barriers to access** As the project develops it is hoped that advertising can be more comprehensive and can look at breaking down some of the barriers identified in the pilot, such as:

  Language/ethnic barriers to certain therapies Links are planned with the NDC Tackling Racism Coordinator to look at ways of reducing barriers and maximising access for black and other minority ethnic groups in the NDC area.

  Crèche facilities Links are planned with the Early Years Project at Barton Hill Settlement.

  Lack of confidence or fear in some local residents to access individual therapy treatments CHIPS plans to develop more group events/self-help workshops across the summer and early autumn in order to attract those local residents who may not be comfortable in accessing the project for one-to-one treatment with a therapist.

Joint work to maximise access for vulnerable groups Plans are under way to work with the following groups: NDC Locks & Bolts Community Safety Project; NDC Older People's Project; NDC School Holiday Activity Programme; NDC Young Women's Project; Fast-track and BEST local employment and business programmes; NDC Tackling Racism Project, reducing racial incidences locally.

(Source: adapted from Monk and Chaplin, 2002)

Comment

1   The report in Box 9.5 is only part of a much more lengthy one. It is not made explicit anywhere in the report what methods were used to evaluate the service. However, the report illustrates that a combination of experimental methods and participatory methods were used: for example, the impact of the therapies on the health of clients was measured using a scale and the report notes that there are case studies of individual people. Many people were treated in this pilot. The report certainly paints an enthusiastic picture of the project, but it may also be necessary to check this general impression against a checklist such as that outlined in Box 9.6 as follows.

■   This report has clear statements of the aims and objectives of each stage of the project and the action research does appear to be entirely relevant to practitioners and users. The participants and stakeholders are clearly described and justified and the local context was considered.

■   The relationship between evaluators and participants was not mentioned in the report but the project itself and the evaluation appear to have been adequately managed.

■   Any ethical issues encountered were not explicitly discussed and the funding for the evaluation itself was not mentioned. However, data were collected in a way that addressed the evaluation issues and this led to clear statements of the findings and outcomes for each phase of the study.

2   So, it may be necessary to conclude that the evaluation report in itself has not enabled you (the putative lottery winner) to decide whether to fund the project. Although the aims seem worthwhile and many positive comments are made, the evidence from the evaluation itself seems patchy or not very clearly thought out. A potential funder would require more definite evidence.

3   Evaluating a project such as this one would require answers to many further questions. For example, what is meant by 'unemployed therapists'? Why are they unemployed? Are they self-employed, registered for professional indemnity and with public liability cover? Or does the project fund these costs as well? What is the cost of paying the therapists and the costs of materials and consumables, laundry, etc.? How are these further costs met? How are the 40 to 50 treatments per week distributed across the different therapies? Was acupressure offered as an independent therapy, or was it part of acupuncture,

shiatsu or reflexology treatments? How is the single therapy room shared between the various therapists? What are the booking arrangements and is there flexibility if there is more demand for some treatments than others? How is the low treatment cost subsidised? What figures are available as evidence?

How were the examples in the project chosen? Are they 'typical' examples? Box 9.5 does not give information about how many different therapies or how many sessions each person attending for treatment received.

Ethical considerations

When conducting an evaluation the following important ethical considerations should always be borne in mind.

The need for ethical approval

The Department of Health's framework for research governance requires all evaluations undertaken in NHS and state-funded social care organisations to obtain ethical approval from an appropriate body. Within the health service, the usual body to approach is the local research ethics committee. Key considerations when applying for approval will be ensuring that the interests of people using the services are fully protected and that they have given their informed consent to taking part. How far evaluation activities are considered to be 'research' for this purpose varies according to the location, subject matter and extent to which people are being required to provide information. Although there is obviously a need for ethical monitoring of any evaluation, sometimes the procedures for obtaining ethics committee approval appear to be unnecessarily complicated and drawn out (Glasziou and Chalmers, 2004).

Bias and credibility

Unless an evaluation has been set up specifically as a self-evaluation, it is generally seen as good practice for the people carrying out the evaluation not to be too intimately involved in the project, or to have strong views on the outcome of the evaluation. This protects the study from bias and helps to maintain an objective perspective. The people conducting the evaluation should also have credibility with the various stakeholders.

Disclosure of potential conflicts of interest

If there are potential conflicts of interest, they should be declared and discussed with the sponsors of the evaluation before the work is begun: for example, if the people doing the evaluation are from an organisation that is competing for funding with the project being evaluated.

Honesty and competence

The people doing the evaluation should be able to demonstrate their competence in carrying out the necessary tasks involved in the evaluation before it starts. Any agreements made should be kept, and total honesty during the data collection, the preparation of the evaluation report and the dissemination of the results are prerequisites.

Ensure the protection of people taking part

This includes ensuring confidentiality and anonymity for people who could be identified in the evaluation, and ensuring that they have given their informed consent to the provision of information. It is important to honour promises of confidentiality and anonymity at all times.

Systematic, accurate and fair evaluation

The evaluation should be as complete and accurate as possible and represent an even-handed search for both the strengths and the weaknesses of the programme being evaluated. Any statistical analysis should be done in an even-handed way, possibly with the assistance of an external specialist.

Show report to interested parties before wide dissemination

A draft of the evaluation report should be shown to the evaluation sponsor and other people who have a thorough knowledge of the project. This should be done in good time so that any changes they suggest can be considered for the final report. However, the final report remains the responsibility of the evaluator.

Waterman et al. (2001) drew up 20 guidelines for assessing quality in evaluation (see Box 9.6). Although these guidelines were developed for all types of evaluation, they can be applied specifically to CAM investigation.

BOX 9.6   GUIDELINES FOR ASSESSING QUALITY IN EVALUATION OF ACTION RESEARCH

1 Is there a clear statement of the aims and objectives of each stage of the research?
2 Was the action research relevant to practitioners and/or users?
3 Were the phases of the project clearly outlined?
4 Were the participants and stakeholders clearly described and justified?
5 Was consideration given to the local context while implementing change?
6 Was the relationship between researchers and participants adequately considered?
7 Was the project managed appropriately?

8   Were ethical issues encountered and how were they dealt with?

9   Was the study adequately funded/supported?

10 Was the length and timetable of the project realistic?

11 Were data collected in a way that addressed the research issue?

12 Were steps taken to promote the rigour of the findings?

13 Were data analyses sufficiently rigorous?

14 Was the study design flexible and responsive?

15 Are there clear statements of the findings and outcomes for each phase of the study?

16 Do the researchers link the data that are presented to their own commentary and interpretation?

17 Is the connection to an existing body of knowledge made clear?

18 Is the extent to which aims and objectives were achieved at each stage discussed?

19 Are the findings transferable?

20 Have the authors articulated the criteria on which their own work is to be read/judged?

(Source: adapted from Waterman et al., 2001, pp. 44–8)

9.7   Conclusion

This chapter described a variety of ways in which CAM projects may be evaluated. To summarise, evaluation is usually considered to be the systematic empirical examination of a social programme or service's design, implementation and impacts, with a view to judging its merit, worth and significance. Evaluation can reduce uncertainty for stakeholders, aid decision making and facilitate service improvement. It may also serve a political function by demonstrating or highlighting certain positive features of the project.

Although this chapter focused on formal types of evaluation, remember that most CAM therapists and people who manage and provide health care facilities are doing their own continuous, informal types of evaluation that are an integral part of reflective practice. A voice within each therapist and CAM service provider should always be asking: 'How am I doing, and could I be doing it any better?' It is also important to recognise that it probably remains impossible to evaluate some imponderables about the healing experience:

> As we seek to refine our research methodologies, we must be ever mindful that the healing encounter likely includes [sic] significant factors that may never be quantifiable.

> (Redwood, 2002, p. 6)

KEY POINTS

- There is no such thing as the 'right' method of research: each project and each situation requires its own ways of considering the relevant questions.

- Evaluation is different from research and audit (although they overlap) and is usually specific to the situation being evaluated.

- Evaluation does not usually produce results that are generalisable or transferable to other situations.

- As the understanding of the complexity of health outcomes grows and develops, so methods of evaluation have evolved and become more refined.

- There are many reasons for doing an evaluation, but it is always necessary to be realistic about what it can achieve.

- All stakeholders should play an active part in the design and dissemination of evaluations and be consulted throughout the process.

- The ethics of the evaluation process should be carefully considered in the design and implementation phases.

- The quality of any evaluation depends on many factors, which the evaluation team should consider.

References

American Evaluation Association (1994) *Guiding Principles for Evaluators: a report of the AEA Task Force on guiding principles for evaluators* [online], www.eval.org/EvaluationDocuments/aeaprin6.html [accessed 26 August 2004].

Barr, A., Hashagen, S. and Taylor, P. (2000) *ABCD Handbook: A Framework for Evaluating Community Development*, London, Community Development Foundation.

Boote, J., Telford, R. and Cooper, C. (2002) 'Consumer involvement in health research: a review and research agenda', *Health Policy*, Vol. 61, No. 2, pp. 213–36.

Carmichael, S. (2003) 'Promoting positive mental health and wellbeing: is there a role for complementary medicine? A study from a patient's perspective', *Health Action Zone Fellowship Report*, Newcastle upon Tyne, Newcastle Primary Care Trust.

Chelimsky, E. (1997) 'Thoughts for a new evaluation society', *Evaluation*, Vol. 3, No. 1, pp. 97–118.

Glasziou, P. and Chalmers, I. (2004) 'Ethics review roulette: what can we learn'?, *British Medical Journal*, Vol. 328, pp. 121–2.

Grabowska, C., Squire, C., MacRae, E. and Robinson, N. (2003) 'Provision of acupuncture in a university health centre: a clinical audit', *Complementary Therapy in Nursing and Midwifery*, Vol. 9, No. 1, pp. 14–19.

INVOLVE (2004) *Promoting Public Involvement in NHS, Public Health and Social Care Research*, Wessex House, Upper Market Street, Eastleigh, Hampshire SO50 9FD.

Monk, J. and Chaplin, S. (2002) *Complementary Health in Partnerships (CHIPS) Evaluation Report – Update*, Bristol, Community at Heart.

Paterson, C. (1996) 'Measuring outcomes in primary care: a patient generated measure, MYMOP, compared with the SF-36 health survey', *British Medical Journal*, Vol. 312, pp. 1016–20.

Quinn Patton, M. (1986) *Utilization Focused Evaluation*, London, Sage Publications.

Redwood, D. (2002) 'Methodological changes in the evaluation of complementary and alternative medicine', *The Journal of Alternative and Complementary Medicine*, Vol. 8, No. 1, pp. 5–6.

Ribeaux, P. and Spence, M. (2001) 'CAM evaluation: what are the research questions?', *Complementary Therapies in Medicine*, Vol. 9, pp. 188–93.

Scriven, M. (1991) *Evaluation Thesaurus* (4th edition), Inverness, CA, Edgepress.

Shadish, W., Cook, T. and Leviton, L. (1991) *Foundations of Program Evaluation: Theories of Practice*, Newbury Park, CA, Sage Publications.

Strauss, A. and Corbin, J. (1990) *Basics of Qualitiative Research: Grounded Theory Procedures and Techniques*, London, Sage Publications.

Telford, R., Chard, J., Dieppe, P., Cooper, C. and Boote, J. (2002) 'Consumer involvement in health research: fact or fiction?', *British Journal of Clinical Governance*, Vol. 7, pp. 92–103.

Thomas, K. and Fitter, M. (2002) 'Possible research strategies for evaluating CAM interventions', in Lewith, G., Jonas, W. B. and Walach, W. (eds) *Clinical Research in Complementary Therapies*, Chapter 4, London, Churchill Livingstone.

Thomas, K., Strong, P. and Luff, D. (2001) *Complementary Medicine Service in a Community Clinic for Patients with Symptoms Associated with the Menopause: Outcome Study and Service Evaluation*, Sheffield, Medical Care Research Unit, University of Sheffield.

Waterman, H., Tillen, D., Dickson, R. and de Koning, K. (2001) 'Action research: a systematic review and guidance for assessment', *Health Technology Assessment*, Vol. 5, No. 23, pp. 43–50.

White, A. and Hart, A. (2002) Editorial: 'Cheap research is likely to be biased', *Complementary Therapies in Medicine*, Vol. 10, pp. 59–60.

Wittmann, W. W. and Walach, H. (2002) 'Evaluating complementary medicine: lessons to be learned from evaluation research', in Lewith, G., Jonas, W. B. and Walach, W. (eds) *Clinical Research in Complementary Therapies*, Chapter 5, London, Churchill Livingstone.

Index